THE GARDENER'S COMPANION TO
MEDICINAL PLANTS

AN A-Z OF HEALING
PLANTS AND HOME
REMEDIES

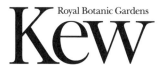
Royal Botanic Gardens
Kew

THE GARDENER'S COMPANION TO

MEDICINAL
PLANTS

AN A-Z OF HEALING
PLANTS AND HOME
REMEDIES

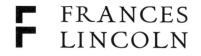
FRANCES
LINCOLN

MONIQUE SIMMONDS,
MELANIE-JAYNE HOWES
AND JASON IRVING

Introduction 6

Plant A-Z 12-217

Recipes

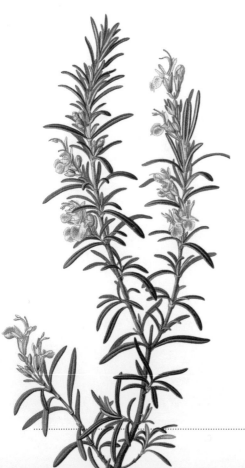

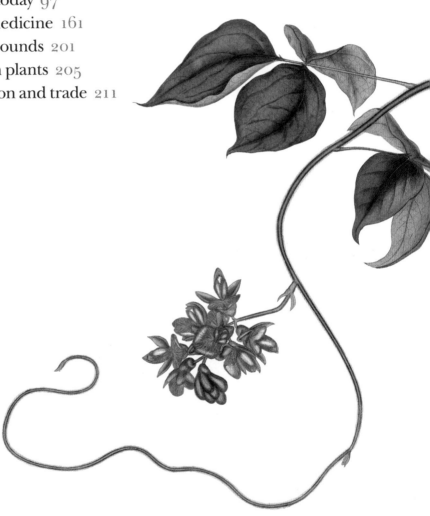

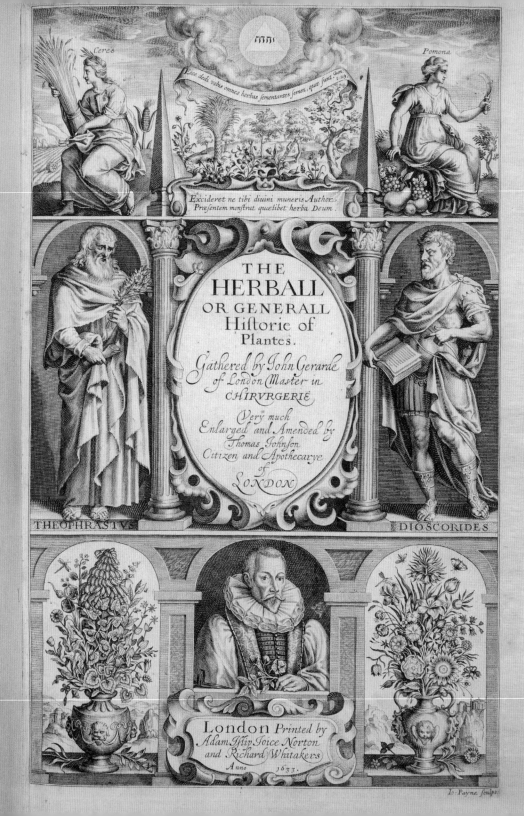

Ceres

Pomona

Hæc dedi vobis omnes herbas sementantes semen, quæ sunt. Gen. 1:29

Excideret ne tibi diuini muneris Author:
Præsentem monstrat quælibet herba Deum.

THE
HERBALL
OR GENERALL
Historie of
Plantes.

Gathered by Iohn Gerarde
of London Master in
CHIRVRGERIE

Very much
Enlarged and Amended by
Thomas Iohnson
Citizen and Apothecarye
of
LONDON

THEOPHRASTVS

DIOSCORIDES

London Printed by
Adam Islip Ioice Norton
and Richard Whitakers
Anno 1633.

Io: Payne. sculp:

Introduction

This book provides gardeners with an overview of plants used in traditional medicine. The ones we have included exhibit a wide range of growing habits, from grasses and flowering plants to shrubs and trees, and come from a wide range of habitats, from sun-baked, rocky hillsides in the Mediterranean to cool, damp boggy soils. You will find aesthetically beautiful plants and others considered to be weeds, but all have medicinal value that we hope may earn them a place in your garden.

From an estimated 300,000 to 400,000 species of terrestrial plants worldwide, 35,500 have a medicinal use. With so many thousands of plants to choose from the criteria for inclusion in this book is that they should have a history of medicinal use and, where possible, to have been the subject of scientific research enabling new medicinal discoveries. The plants must also have been used for a wide range of medical conditions. Notable omissions are plants that are already well-known through pharmaceutical research, such as the Madagascar periwinkle (*Catharanthus roseus*), foxglove (*Digitalis purpurea*) and the yew tree (*Taxus baccata*).

Prior to the twentieth century, medicinal plants were the main resource for western health care. While there has been a recent resurgence in interest in them in the west, in Africa, South America and Asia plants have, and still play, a key role in primary health care. To use medicinal plants appropriately, it is important that we have a better understanding about their safety and efficacy. Without that knowledge, we cannot provide reliable information about which plants offer the most benefits, and which plants can or cannot be used in combination with other plants or with modern pharmaceutical drugs. As we increase our knowledge about diseases, there is a better understanding of how many of the medicinal plants could, if used appropriately, alleviate some of the symptoms associated with different health conditions.

The main A to Z reference section in the book lists 277 plants, each entry is illustrated and gives a short description of the plant. These provide an insight into the wonderful diversity of medicinal plants. The Latin binomial name for each plant is given – genus followed by species – along with the common name and the parts of the plant that are used for medicinal purposes. In the 'Traditional uses' and 'Medicinal discoveries' sections, we provide a taste of old and new information. 'Traditional uses' explains how the plants were and are used in Europe, the Americas and Asia. It includes quotes from some of the early herbalists including John Gerard

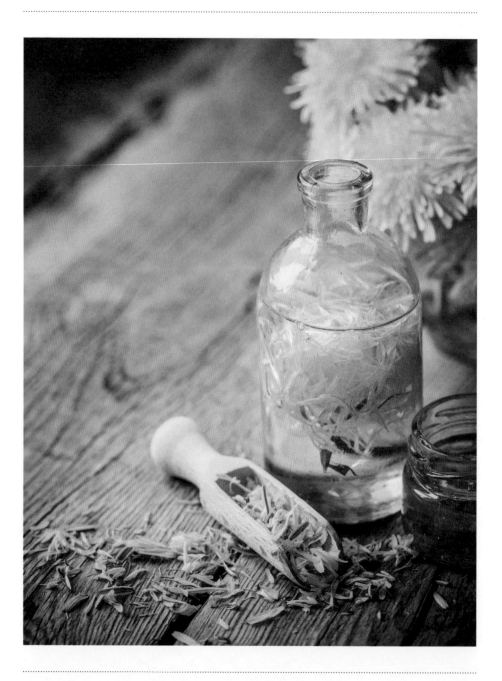

and Nicholas Culpeper (seventeenth century). The 'Medicinal discoveries' section provides a summary of scientific findings about actual or potential medicinal uses. In some cases the findings can explain why the plant could be useful for different ailments, but, generally, there is a lack of clinical data from studies in humans to fully validate these claims. We also detail the compounds in some of the plants that might be responsible for the medicinal properties of the plant or contribute to its use.

Twenty-four plants have been given a more detailed entry and an easy-to-follow recipe so you can make your own plant-based remedies. The plants were chosen because of their well-documented tradition of use.

There are additional features in this book that look at the modern uses of herbal medicines as well as the different types of traditional medicine systems, such as those used in China and India. We also provide an overview of the importance of conserving plants, the role of some of the compounds that occur in plants, and of the importance of plants in discovering new drugs.

Throughout the book there are references to a few notable early herbalists, including John Gerard and Nicholas Culpeper. You will find an overview of the role these men played in collating information about the medicinal uses of plants on page 81.

Flowers of dandelion (*Taraxacum officinale*) infusing in water to make a syrup with honey.

Remedies: using the recipes

We wanted to give you an idea of the possibilities for using plants from your garden as herbal remedies. We also wanted to show you how to make teas, tinctures, oils and creams. The twenty-four recipes in the book are each designed to give you a broad overview of the many different preparations employed in herbal medicine. They are simple to prepare – you need only basic cooking skills. Note that while the recipes are particularly suited to the plant being used, the plant in the recipe can be prepared in many other ways.

The quantities used in the recipes are for making small amounts of each remedy, but if you want to scale up production simply increase the proportions of each ingredient by an equal amount.

Making herbal remedies at home

Most of the recipes require dried plant material. This is because plants contain around seventy per cent water which will dilute the extract and can make it more susceptible to spoiling. Step-by-step instructions on drying herbs and roots are given on page 207. Once an extract is made the plant material is removed, making it easier to take and reducing the risk of spoiling. Straining through muslin will filter out any small bits of plant.

Many of the kitchen utensils you need are the same as those used in jam making: bowls, sauce pans, spoons, scales, clean squares of muslin, kitchen funnel, assorted jars and bottles with an airtight seal for storing. Utensils should be clean and dry and bottles and jars should be sterilized before use.

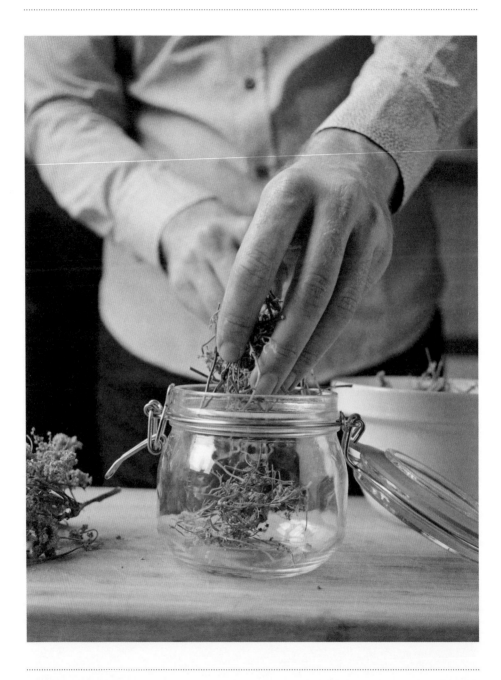

Most of the ingredients you will find in your garden or in your local shops. A few of the recipes require more specialist ingredients and equipment but, fortunately, these are now widely available on the internet.

Ideally, both dried herbs and herbal remedies, such as tinctures and syrups, should be stored in airtight containers that protect them from sunlight to preserve them for as long as possible. Dark glass jars are ideal, but if the remedy is in regular use then a clear jar will do as it will be used up quickly.

As the oils and creams in this book will be homemade and, therefore, won't include the many preservatives that may go into over-the-counter herbal medicines or cosmetics, they are more vulnerable to spoiling and have a shorter shelf life. To keep them fresh for longer, store them in the fridge and/or add vitamin E as a preservative.

All remedies should be labelled with the ingredients listed and date of preparation – it is very easy to forget what that strange smelling liquid is at the back of your cupboard!

Using the herbal remedies in this book

The twenty-four remedies in this book have a long tradition of safe use. However, different people may react differently to a plant, so only use a small amount – and only once – when trying a plant for the first time. For example, a small number of people are allergic to plants of the daisy family (Asteraceae), which can cause an allergic response, such as itchy skin, rash and nausea. With an internal medicine try a single dose and wait for at least a day to see if there is any unusual effect. With remedies applied externally (topically), always do a patch test by rubbing the cream or oil on a small area and waiting several hours to see if any reaction occurs. The doses described in this book have been given for an average healthy adult. Pay attention to how a remedy is affecting you throughout the time you take it and if you suspect anything is wrong then stop taking it and seek medical advice from a health professional. Always get medical advice if the symptoms are serious and/or persistent. If you are pregnant, breastfeeding, have a medical condition or are taking any medication then check with a health professional before using the remedies in this book.

This book is not a medical manual and is not intended as a guide to self-diagnosis and self-treatment.

Adding dried meadowsweet flowers (*Filipendula ulmaria*) to a jar to make a tincture (see page 83 for the recipe).

Achillea millefolium
Yarrow

Achillea is named after Achilles, the hero of Greek mythology, who used yarrow to treat his soldiers when they were wounded in battle. It has been known as *herba militaris* in Latin and woundwort in English. Old herbals often include recipes for yarrow ointment as it was valued for its use in staunching bleeding. Perhaps because of this property it was also employed to reduce excessive menstruation and painful periods.

Yarrow was one of the many herbs that were added to beer before hops came to dominate brewing. These plants served a dual purpose, preserving the beer by inhibiting microbes and adding bitterness to what would otherwise be a relatively flavourless drink. This points to the antibacterial action of yarrow, which would be of use in wound healing.

There is very little scientific research into the effects of yarrow, which contrasts sharply with the almost endless list of traditional uses for the plant. It is recommended for varicose veins, weak digestion, gut spasm, haemorrhoids, diarrhoea, urinary tract infections, colds, allergies, to break fever and liver problems.

Grow Native to temperate regions of the northern hemisphere, this perennial is found in lawns where it spreads to form a dense mat. Flowering stems can grow to a height of 50 cm (20 inch). Yarrow prefers full sun but will grow in most soils so long as they are well drained.
Harvest Leaves can be gathered year round and will regrow quickly. The clusters of aromatic flowers appear from early spring to late autumn.
Caution May cause allergic reactions, such as dermatitis, in anyone sensitive to plants of the daisy (Asteraceae) family.

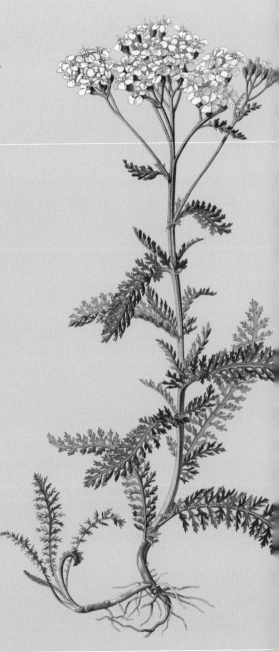

Yarrow glycerin

Glycerin is a useful extraction for those who cannot take alcohol, and the sweetness helps mask any bitter flavours. A glycerin prepared from yarrow flowers is traditionally used to aid digestion and ease the symptoms of hayfever, colds and flu. Take 5 ml (1 teaspoon) in water twice a day.

30 heads of yarrow flowers (fresh or dry)

200 ml (7 fl oz) water

400 ml (14 fl oz) vegetable glycerin

You will also need: saucepan; scissors; measuring jug; sterilized wide-necked jar with lid; square of muslin; funnel; sterilized bottle with stopper

1. Snip the flower heads into small pieces using scissors. Put in a saucepan, pour over the water and heat gently with the lid on for five minutes. Remove from the heat and leave to stand for half an hour with the lid on, then pour into the jar.

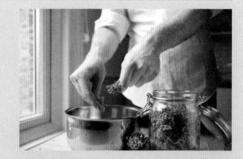

2. Pour the glycerin into the jar and stir to combine. Leave for two weeks in the fridge, giving the jar a good shake every few days.

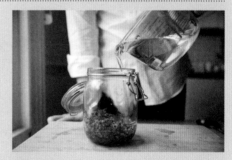

3. Strain through a muslin-lined funnel into a sterilized bottle. Store in the fridge for up to a year.

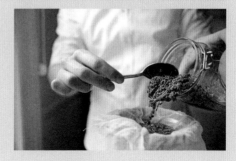

Acanthus mollis
Bear's breech

Herbaceous perennial producing white flowers with deep purple bracts. Grows in southern Europe and N.W. Africa.

Part(s) used Leaf.
Traditional uses Reputed to purify the blood and reduce fevers. Preparations were applied to treat and clean wounds; they were also believed to strengthen joints and restore broken bones. In Italy, the leaves were used for skin diseases such as psoriasis.
Medicinal discoveries In laboratory studies, leaf extracts show some anti-inflammatory properties; however, more research is needed to discover any biological activities that might explain the traditional or potential uses.

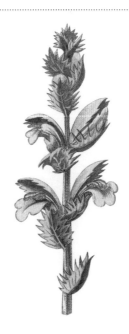

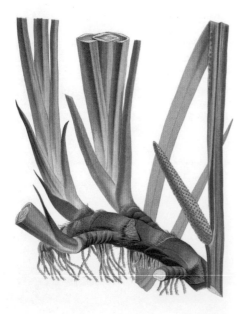

Acorus calamus
Sweet flag

Native to Asia, different varieties are found throughout Europe and the Americas. It is a wetland plant that grows by the side of lakes and streams.

Part(s) used Leaf, rhizome.
Traditional uses Fragrant sweet flag has a long tradition as a medicinal plant: it is mentioned in early Persian texts and is thought to be the 'calamus' (the sweet cane of Palestine) of the Old Testament. It was used to treat fevers and eye problems.
Medicinal discoveries The plant's essential oils are used for anorexia, colic and chronic dyspepsia. Scientific studies can explain the oil's use in alleviating dyspepsia and colic.

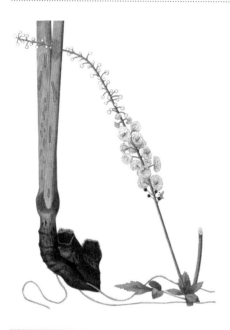

Actaea racemosa
Black cohosh

N. American herbaceous perennial with small white flowers.

Part(s) used Rhizome, root.
Traditional uses Used to alleviate rheumatic complaints and to treat tinnitus, uterine spasms and menstrual pain. Reputed to have sedative and cough-relieving properties, it has been used as a remedy for whooping cough.
Medicinal discoveries Current interest in the plant has focused on its potential to relieve menopausal symptoms. Clinical studies, however, have not been conclusive and further research is needed to determine possible benefits and therapeutic effects. There have been concerns that it might cause liver disorders.

Aesculus hippocastanum
Horse chestnut

Native to the Balkan Peninsular, horse chestnut trees are now found growing in deciduous and mixed woodlands in many parts of Europe. It is also planted as an ornamental street tree.

Part(s) used Bark, flower, leaf, seed.
Traditional uses Extracts from the leaves, flowers and seeds were used to treat rheumatism, haemorrhoids and circulation problems. The bark was used as a tonic, to treat fevers and external ulcers.
Medicinal discoveries Seeds contain a compound called aescin and flavonoids. In controlled clinical studies, these compounds have been shown to treat the symptoms associated with varicose veins.

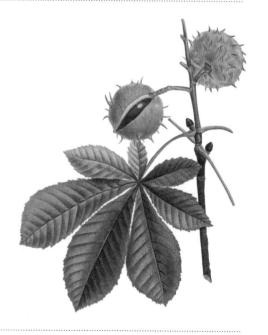

Agrimonia eupatoria
Agrimony

A herbaceous perennial plant with
spikes of yellow flowers found growing
in hedgerows and grasslands in Europe,
Asia and N. Africa.

Part(s) used Flowering aerial parts, root.
Traditional uses In medieval times it was
used as a poultice for treating wounds in
people as well as animals, and made into an
infusion to treat dysentery and diarrhoea.
Dioscorides mentions its use in treating liver
complaints. More recently it has been widely
used as a tonic and diuretic for treating
sore throats, colds and coughs. The roots
were used to treat fevers and the flowering
aerial parts to treat many digestive disorders
including nausea and bad breath. Roots
and dry leaves were used to treat bladder
and kidney problems, worm infestation,
diabetes, and ruptured blood vessels.
Medicinal discoveries Studies have shown
extracts have antibacterial properties,
which could explain its use for mild
diarrhoea, as a gargle to treat throat
infections and to support wound healing.
A small clinical trial that involved an
infusion of agrimony supported its
traditional use in treating skin ailments.
The patients that took the infusion also
showed improvements in their general
health. It contains high levels of
tannins which contribute to
its astringent properties.

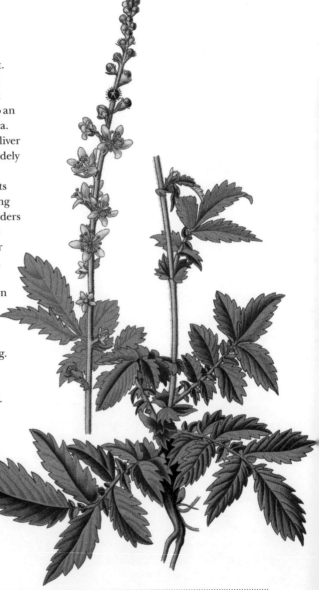

Ajuga reptans
Bugle

Native to Europe, this blue-flowering perennial is a good groundcover plant for shade in damp, neutral or acid soils.

Part(s) used Aerial parts.
Traditional uses In the Middle Ages bugle was regarded as a 'cure-all' plant with a diverse range of uses. Today, although it has fallen out of use, bugle retains a reputation as a wound-healing plant, as a treatment for diarrhoea and as a gargle to soothe a sore throat.
Medicinal discoveries Currently under investigation for its use in treating wounds and bruises.

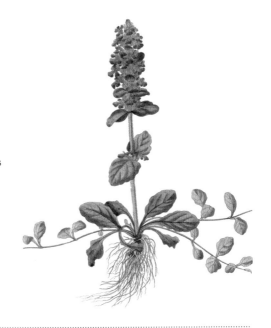

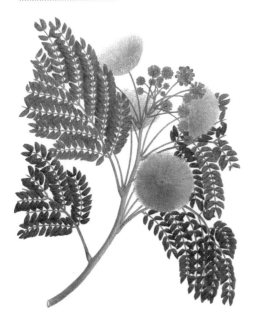

Albizia julibrissin
Silk tree

Large shrub or small tree with fern-like leaves and clusters of fluffy pink flowers. Grows in tropical and subtropical regions.

Part(s) used Bark, flower.
Traditional uses In traditional Chinese medicine bark was used as a sedative and for trauma. It was reputed to have astringent and diuretic properties, and to stimulate the circulation and uterus. Flowers were believed to have sedative properties and to alleviate indigestion.
Medicinal discoveries Scientific studies have revealed that chemical constituents of the flowers might have sedative properties, while bark preparations have been investigated for potential to alleviate anxiety and depression.

Alchemilla xanthochlora
Lady's mantle

Perennial herb found growing throughout Europe and N. America in neutral or chalky grasslands, on river banks and in woodlands. A popular garden plant for the front of the border, with frothy sprays of small yellow flowers in summer. Its kidney-shaped leaves hold drops of water after rain.

Part(s) used Flowering aerial parts, root.

Traditional uses The flowering aerial parts were reputed to alleviate female disorders such as menstrual irregularities and menopausal symptoms. Said to have astringent properties, the root was used to treat diarrhoea and to stop wounds from bleeding. The herbalist Nicholas Culpeper (see page 81) claimed it was, 'very proper for inflamed wounds and to stay bleeding, vomitings, fluxes of all sorts, bruises by falls and ruptures', and that it, 'quickly healeth green wounds'. Leaves were reputed to treat spasms and convulsions. It was believed that if the herb was placed under the pillow at night it would aid sleep.

Medicinal discoveries There has been interest in the use of lady's mantle to control irregular menstrual bleeding, and some small studies suggest positive effects, although more clinical studies in humans are needed to conclude any benefits. Laboratory tests suggest the plant has anti-inflammatory and wound-healing properties. It has also undergone assessment for its potential to heal mouth ulcers.

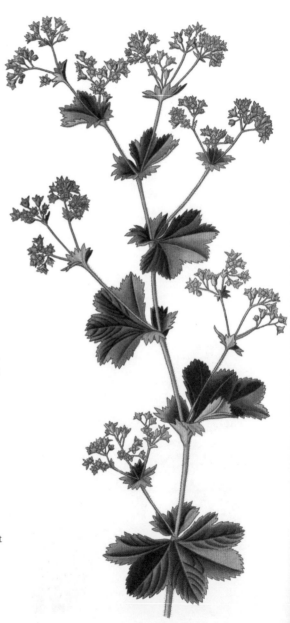

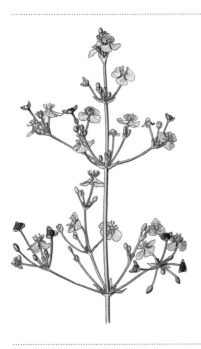

Alisma plantago-aquatica
Water-plantain

Perennial found growing in shallow, fresh water throughout Europe, N. Africa and Australia. It produces small white to pale purple flowers in summer.

Part(s) used Leaf, root.
Traditional uses The roots of water-plantain were recommended as a cure for rabies, while its leaves were used to treat cystitis, dysentery and digestive disorders. Homeopaths have used it as a remedy for gastric disorders.
Medicinal discoveries Scientific studies have shown that extracts from the roots and leaves have antibacterial activity, can lower blood pressure and might protect the liver.

Alliaria petiolata
Garlic mustard, Jack-by-the-hedge

A biennial found in a wide range of habitats in temperate climates, including Britain. It grows best in moist, fertile soils. In N. America it is considered an invasive species.

Part(s) used Aerial parts.
Traditional uses Used to treat a wide range of infections and wounds and to improve poor circulation.
Medicinal discoveries Garlic mustard is related to the onion. It contains a group of compounds called allyl isothiocyanates which have antiseptic and anti-inflammatory properties that could explain its traditional uses. It is also a rich source of vitamin C.

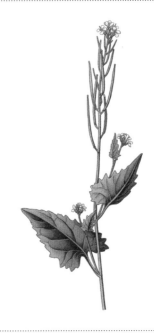

Allium sativum
Garlic

The Roman natural philosopher Pliny the Elder recommended garlic for more than sixty different health problems, including mixed with honey for dog and serpents' bites, in vinegar for bruises, for toothache, asthma, hoarseness, skin eruptions, jaundice and tumours. Pliny wrote that garlic 'clears the arteries and opens the veins'. Research shows it can lower blood pressure and high cholesterol levels and so reduce the risk of heart problems.

Garlic's powerful antimicrobial action explains many of its traditional uses against respiratory, intestinal and skin infections. An old English herbal from the ninth century, Bald's *Leechbook*, contains a recipe for an eye salve made of garlic, onion or leeks, wine and cow bile. When this preparation was tested against the 'super bug' methicillin-resistant *Staphylococcus aureus*, it killed ninety per cent of the bacteria – a significant result as the strain was resistant to most antibiotics.

The notorious garlic breath is thought to have a beneficial effect on many respiratory infections as the antibacterial compounds pass through the airways. The pungent sulphur compounds that are mostly responsible for its medicinal actions break down on heating so it is best taken raw.

Grow Native to Central Asia and N.E. Iran, garlic has been widely cultivated for thousands of years. Plant individual cloves in late autumn or early spring in fertile, well-drained soil that gets plenty of sun.
Harvest Lift when foliage starts to yellow. To dry, leave in a cool, airy place for two to four weeks.
Caution Anyone taking anticoagulants or with a blood clotting disorder should use with caution.

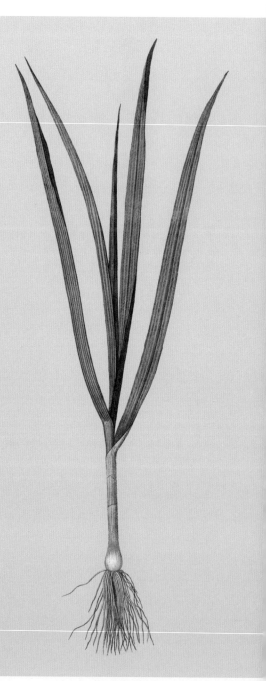

Garlic oxymel

If you can't stomach eating garlic raw, this recipe will make it more palatable. Honey and vinegar are both valued for their medicinal and preservative actions: mixed together they make an ancient remedy called an oxymel. When you have an infection, take one teaspoon three times a day.

150 g (5 oz) honey

150 ml (5 fl oz) cider vinegar

1 bulb garlic

2 teaspoons (5 g/0.2 oz) aniseed seeds

You will also need: scales; sterilized jar with lid; measuring jug; garlic crusher; pestle and mortar; fine sieve; sterilized bottle with stopper

1. Measure the honey into an empty jar on scales. Pour in the vinegar and stir to combine.

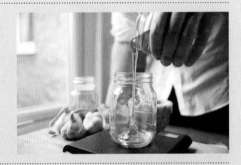

2. Peel and crush the garlic, grind the seeds with a pestle and mortar and add them to the honey and vinegar mixture. Stir to combine and pop the lid on the jar.

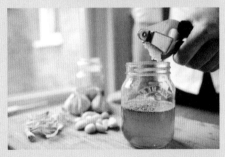

3. Leave the mixture for one week in the fridge. Once a day give the jar a good shake. After a week, strain the mixture through a fine sieve into a sterilized bottle. Will keep for six months in the fridge.

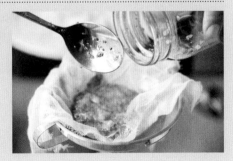

Aloe vera
Aloe

This short-stemmed succulent has green fleshy leaves that taper to sharp tips. There are also short spines along the leaf margins. Originally from the Arabian Peninsula, aloe is now grown commercially worldwide. It needs a light sandy soil and plenty of sun – it would do well in a rockery. It is frost-tender.

Part(s) used Leaf.

Traditional uses The leaf cells are filled with a clear gel that exudes from the plant when cut. This was used in ointments to treat wounds, burns, eczema, psoriasis and a range of other skin conditions. The plant has also been used as a laxative.

Medicinal discoveries Extensive laboratory and clinical studies have shown that aloe extracts can help alleviate bronchial asthma and mouth ulcers. Leaf-gel preparations have anti-inflammatory properties that may help arthritic conditions. When homogenized, aloe has exhibited anti-diabetic properties. The gel is antibacterial and acts as a protective barrier – both properties that confirm its traditional use in treating skin disorders.

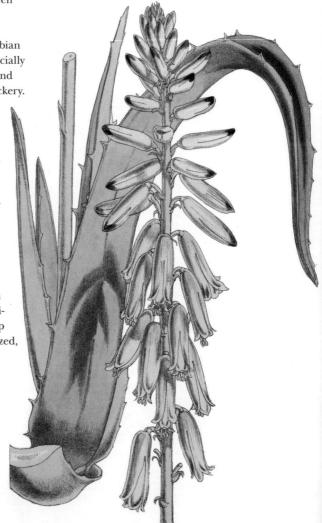

Aloysia citrodora
Lemon verbena

A lemon-scented, deciduous shrub with pale to mid-green leaves and lilac-white flowers. Native to N. and S. America, it is popular as a garden and house plant.

Part(s) used Flower, leaf.

Traditional uses Reputed to have a calming effect and to aid sleep, lemon verbena was also used to reduce gut spasms, aid digestion and to treat diarrhoea and flatulence. It was thought to alleviate asthma, cold and flu symptoms and reduce fevers. Preparations were reputed to stimulate the skin.

Medicinal discoveries The essential oil from the leaves is used in aromatherapy and in perfumery. It has also been investigated for its potential effects relevant to Alzheimer's disease. Scientific studies revealed that components of the oil can bind to receptors on nerve cells that are considered important for memory and that the oil had protective effects on nerve cells. Other species of *Aloysia* and their constituents have been of interest for their potential to relieve anxiety and depression, although more research is needed to determine any possible benefits.

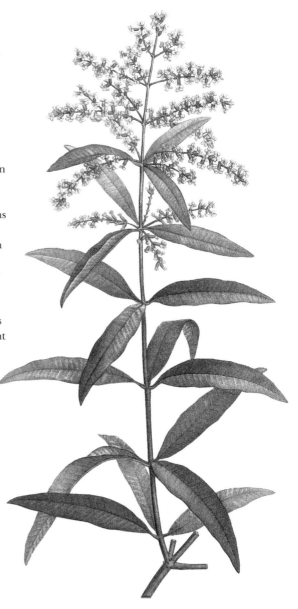

Althaea officinalis
Marshmallow

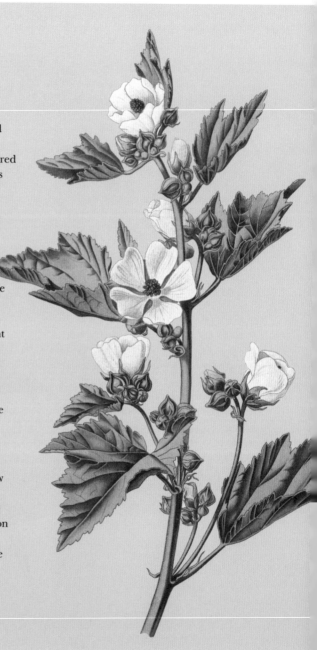

Say marshmallow and most people will think of the sweet and be surprised to discover that a plant shares the name. It was the root of the marshmallow that was originally used to prepare throat and cough lozenges, a practice that has been traced back to ancient Egypt. The powdered root is mucilaginous, meaning it contains carbohydrates that bind well with water to form a sticky viscous substance. This property helps it bind together with other powdered herbs to form lozenges, and soothes by coating inflamed mucous membranes.

It is used to calm an itchy throat, to soothe an infected urinary tract and to coat the lining of an inflamed digestive tract, providing a more favourable environment for good bacteria. Poultices of the roots or leaves are used externally as a drawing poultice and to soothe inflammation. Marshmallow was thought to act via a reflex action on the lungs, resulting in the loosening of mucus. The lozenges were given for asthma, bronchitis, hoarseness, coughs and colds.

Grow As the name suggests, marshmallow thrives in boggy conditions, although it is also well suited to drier coastal areas. The pale pink flowers appear in late summer on stems up to 1.5 m (5 ft). Prefers full sun.
Harvest The root is ready to harvest in the second year of growth after flowering.

Marshmallow lozenges

This preparation is similar to the lozenges traditionally used to treat sore throats and acid reflux. Pop one in the mouth and slowly suck; take several a day as required.

100 g (3½ oz) dried marshmallow root

30 g (1 oz) dried liquorice root

3 tablespoons honey

You will also need: scales; spice grinder; bowls; sieve; tablespoon; small saucepan; cooling rack; airtight storage tin; greaseproof paper

1. Grind the marshmallow root into a fine powder using a spice grinder. Transfer to a small, clean bowl, sifting to remove any lumps. Repeat with the liquorice root. In a fresh bowl, mix together 3 tablespoons marshmallow powder and 1 tablespoon liquorice powder.

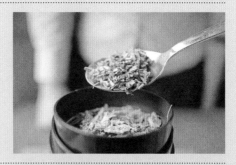

2. Gently warm the honey in a small pan until runny then trickle over the measured powders. Keep stirring and checking the consistency – stop adding honey if the mixture starts to get too moist. If you need to dry it out a bit add a little more of the powdered roots.

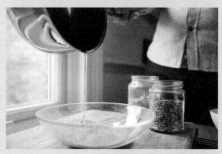

3. Transfer the remaining powders to a bowl. Using your hands, take small pieces of the honey mixture and roll it into small balls. Roll each ball in the powder, then lay out to dry on a cooling rack with space in between until hard. Store in an airtight tin layered between sheets of greaseproof paper.

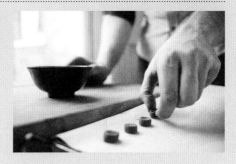

Ammi visnaga
Toothpick weed

Native to Asia but now found across Europe and N. Africa. Often grown as a cut-flower for its dense clusters of white-green flowers in summer. Grows in full sun, in neutral, well-drained soils.

Part(s) used Flower stalk, fruit.
Traditional uses Fruiting rays of the flower stalks are sold in N. Africa as toothpicks. The seed was used to treat colic, kidney stones and urinary problems.
Medicinal discoveries A compound from the plant called khellin was isolated and then synthesized to develop the drug amiodarone, which is used to treat irregular heartbeats.

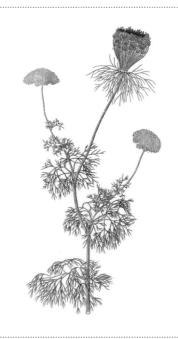

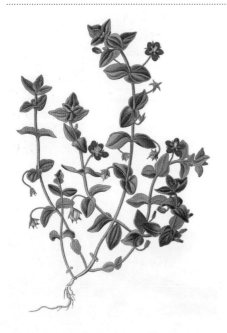

Anagallis arvensis
Scarlet pimpernel

Native to temperate parts of Europe, W. Asia and N. Africa. The plant has small orange-red flowers and is found growing in neutral and alkaline soils in open areas. If not contained it can be invasive.

Part(s) used Aerial parts.
Traditional uses It was reported to have a wide range of uses including a 'remedy for the bites of mad dogs and to dispel sadness'. It was called *Anagallis* by Dioscorides, which is from the Greek *anagelao*, 'to laugh,' because it relieved depression.
Medicinal discoveries Currently being researched for its antiviral properties.

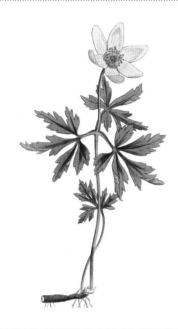

Anemone nemorosa
Wood anemone, wind-flower

Pretty, low-growing, creeping perennial found growing in European woods. In late spring it produces white or pink flowers.

Part(s) used Leaf, root.
Traditional uses The herbalist Nicholas Culpeper (see page 81) claimed that a leaf decoction 'cures the leprosy', and that the juice 'snuffed up the nose purgeth the head mightily'. The root 'bringeth away many watery and phlegmatic humours and is therefore excellent for the lethargy'. *Anemone raddeana* is a traditional Chinese medicine for rheumatism and inflammation of veins.
Medicinal discoveries Scientific studies have shown it has antibacterial properties. *A. raddeana* has potential anticancer effects.

Anethum graveolens
Dill

Thought to originate from S.W. Asia and India, this tall-growing, aniseed-scented annual has feathery leaves and yellow flowers. Plant in well-drained soils in full sun. Hardy.

Part(s) used Leaf, seed.
Traditional uses Dill is used as a culinary herb and as a traditional medicine for the treatment of jaundice, headache, boils, nausea, lack of appetite, stomach and liver problems.
Medicinal discoveries Gripe water is a formulation that contains the essential oil from dill seeds. However, although it is still given to infants to treat colic and wind there is very little scientific data to support this use.

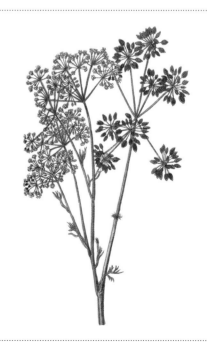

Angelica archangelica
Angelica

A tall-growing, aromatic biennial that occurs in N. and E. Europe. It produces big, rounded umbels of green-yellow flowers on long stems. Prefers a moist loamy soil in full or partial shade. Grown as a culinary herb.

Part(s) used Fruit, leaf, root.

Traditional uses In medieval times, angelica was named the angelic herb as it was believed to protect against evil and cure all ills. Reputed to have expectorant properties, it was used for coughs, colds, pleurisy and bronchitis. It was also used to increase sweating and reduce fevers, including typhus fever. An infusion prepared from the root was a remedy for flatulence, indigestion and general debility. The stems were used for a feeble stomach and juice from the stems and root was a remedy for rheumatism and gout. An infusion of the leaves was regarded as a 'healthful, strengthening tonic'. The sixteenth-century herbalist John Gerard (see page 81) claimed angelica 'cureth the bitings of mad dogs and all other venomous beasts'.

Medicinal discoveries Although angelica has many traditional uses these have not been extensively explored in scientific studies. Some laboratory investigations suggest angelica has antibacterial and antifungal properties and can modulate muscle spasms. A compound isolated from angelica called bergapten has been used in combination with ultraviolet light irradiation therapy in the treatment of psoriasis. Some individuals may experience dermatitis following contact with angelica if their skin is exposed to sunlight.

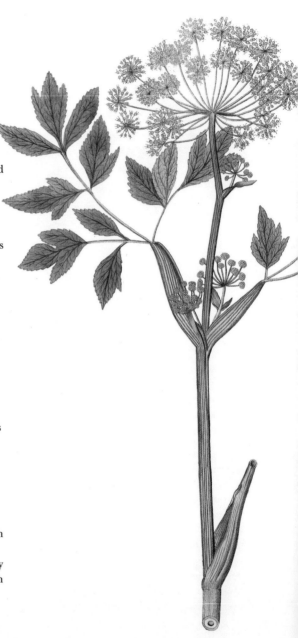

Apium graveolens
Wild celery

Biennial or short-lived perennial herb with bulbous root that grows by the coast in temperate areas of Europe, Africa and Asia. Smells strongly of celery.

Part(s) used Whole plant.
Traditional uses The plant has been used to treat a range of conditions including high blood pressure, indigestion, sleeplessness, urinary infections, nervous conditions, rheumatism, arthritis and kidney problems.
Medicinal discoveries Extracts from the fruit have been shown to have antiseptic and anti-inflammatory properties which could explain its use for rheumatism, arthritis, gout and urinary tract infections.

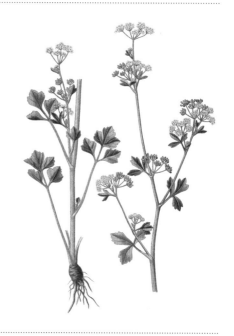

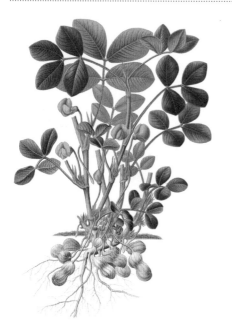

Arachis hypogaea
Peanut, groundnut

Annual legume with spreading stems and small yellow flowers that develop into pods. Native to S. America.

Part(s) used Seed, seed oil.
Traditional uses Cultivated since ancient times in S. America for use in sacred ceremonies, for decorations and as a tonic.
Medicinal discoveries An important food and oil crop that is used in the production of some cooking fats and peanut butter. The oil is obtained by crushing the seeds and is used to formulate some nutritional therapies. It is also used as an enema to soften stools in constipation, in drops to soften ear wax and in emollient creams for the skin.

Arctium lappa
Burdock, greater burdock

Tall, upright biennial, native to Europe, which produces purple, thistle-like flowers, followed by fruits with hooked spines.

Part(s) used   Root, seed, leaf.

Traditional uses   An old English name for burdock was *reafe*, meaning 'robber', referring to the burrs that seize wool from sheep as they pass by. The herbalist Nicholas Culpeper (see page 81) described burdock as 'Happy major', and claimed that 'the leaves applied to places troubled with the shrinking in the sinews or arteries give much ease', and that the leaf or root juice 'given to drink with old wine doth wonderfully help the biting of any serpents'. The root mixed with salt was applied to 'helpeth those that are bit by a mad dog', and the seed 'being drunk in wine doth wonderfully help the sciatica'. Roots were a remedy for boils, scurvy and rheumatic complaints and leaves were applied as a poultice to swellings and to the feet for 'hysterical disorders'.

Medicinal discoveries   According to scientific studies, the roots, leaves and flowers have antimicrobial properties. There is a suggestion that the roots and leaves might have a diuretic effect and can also lower blood glucose levels. These actions have not yet been confirmed in clinical studies. Burdock has been investigated for anticancer properties and the seeds have been of interest to alleviate dry skin conditions.

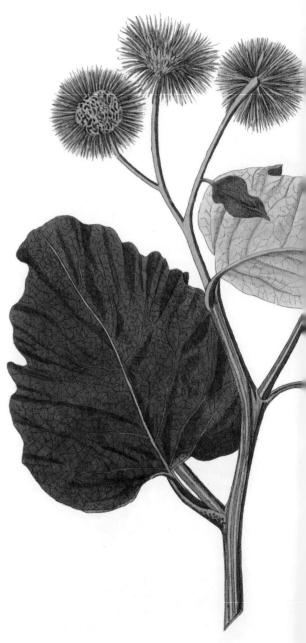

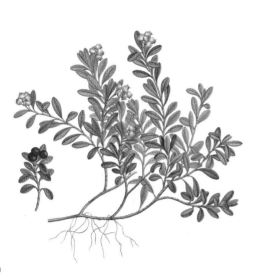

Arctostaphylos uva-ursi
Bearberry, uva-ursi

Rapid-growing evergreen shrub that occurs on heaths in Northern Europe and America, and parts of Asia. Produces white and pink flowers followed by red fruits.

Part(s) used Leaf.
Traditional uses Used from the twelfth century by the Welsh 'Physicians of Myddfai' as an infusion for kidney and bladder diseases. It was reputed to treat urine infections and inflammation, and was used as a diuretic.
Medicinal discoveries In scientific studies bearberry has shown antimicrobial and anti-inflammatory properties. More research is needed to understand its potential benefits in alleviating urine infections in humans.

Armoracia rusticana
Horseradish

Upright, herbaceous perennial that occurs in parts of Europe with small white flowers. Can be invasive. Widely used in a sauce to accompany roast beef.

Part(s) used Root.
Traditional uses Horseradish was used to stimulate digestion, as an expectorant and it was also believed to treat dropsy and scurvy. The herbalist Culpeper (see page 81) claimed that,'if bruised and laid to a part grieved with gout, sciatica, joint ache or hard swellings of the spleen or liver, it doth wonderfully help them all'. It was also used to treat intestinal worms.
Medicinal discoveries Horseradish may have anti-inflammatory properties.

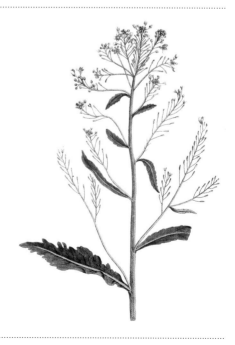

Arnica montana
Arnica, leopard's bane

A herbaceous, alpine perennial that occurs in Europe. This aromatic plant produces yellow daisy-like flowers from midsummer to autumn and would make an attractive addition to a rock garden.

Part(s) used Flower.

Traditional uses Arnica tincture was applied to sprains, bruises and wounds, and was also used as a remedy for unbroken chilblains. Occasionally taken as a stimulant, to combat fevers and as a diuretic, it was also used for heart complaints such as angina. Arnica was prepared as a foot-bath for tender feet and applied to the scalp to stimulate hair growth. Other traditional uses included treating mouth inflammations, such as gingivitis, and to alleviate insect bites.

Medicinal discoveries Some small clinical studies suggested that when arnica preparations are applied to the limbs they may reduce muscle aches and improve vein tone, fluid retention and the feeling of heaviness in the legs. It has also been of interest for alleviating joint stiffness and pains, and for bruises and burns when applied to the skin. Arnica can be poisonous if taken internally, and may cause dermatitis in some individuals if used on the skin.

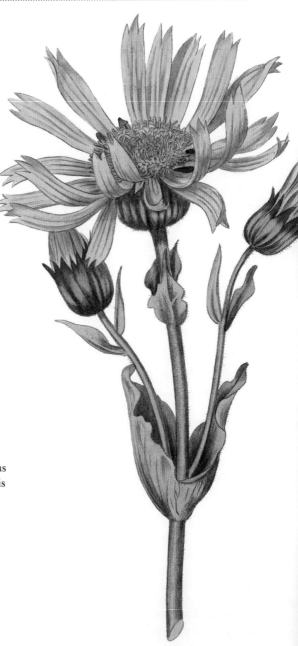

Artemisia annua
Sweet wormwood

A native of Asia, this shrub-like annual herb is now found growing in most temperate parts of the world. Likes full sun and a well-drained soil. It has aromatic leaves and small yellow-green flowers in late summer. *Artemisia annua* has green leaves, whereas *A. abrotanum* and *A. absinthium* have attractive grey-green foliage.

Part(s) used Flowering aerial parts.

Traditional uses In traditional Chinese medicine *A. annua* was used to treat fevers (as were most wormwoods). The ash of *A. abrotanum* was used by boys to promote the growth of a beard, whereas *A. absinthium* was used to restore mental functions and treat stomach and throat infections.

Medicinal discoveries In 1972, the compound artemisinin was isolated from *A. annua* and shown to have antimalarial activity. Artemisinin was developed into an antimalarial drug with the support of the World Health Organization. The Chinese scientist Youyou Tu who was involved in the initial research on the plant shared the 2015 Nobel Prize in Physiology and Medicine.

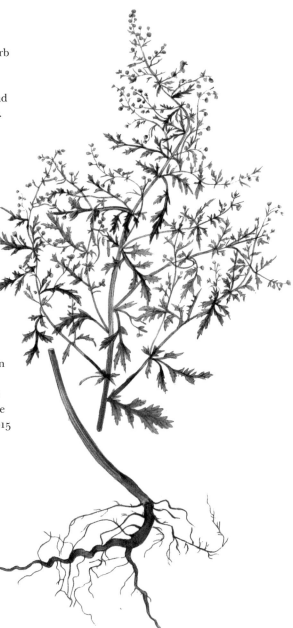

Asparagus officinalis
Asparagus

European perennial that is widely grown as a seasonal vegetable. The plant has upright stems with bell-shaped, green-white flowers.

Part(s) used Tuber-like root, young shoot.
Traditional uses Considered to have restorative and cleansing properties, asparagus was given as a diuretic and to treat urine infections. It was also said to be good for treating rheumatism, gout and constipation.
Medicinal discoveries Asparagus has been investigated for its potential use in controlling diabetes and high cholesterol. Laboratory studies suggest it may have blood glucose and cholesterol-lowering effects. It may also have anticancer properties.

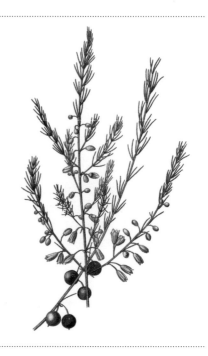

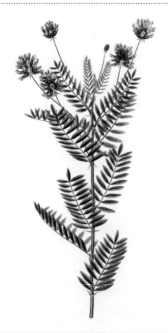

Astragalus mongholicus
Milk vetch

Perennial that occurs in eastern Asia and produces yellow flowers and large pods.

Part(s) used Root.
Traditional uses A traditional Chinese medicine, often formulated with other herbs, to treat poor circulation and low energy. Also taken for skin eruptions and kidney disorders. Thought to boost the immune system and combat allergies and colds.
Medicinal discoveries Modern interest has focused on its potential to treat kidney disease. Clinical studies in humans suggest that when combined with conventional medicines, milk vetch might have some benefits as a kidney treatment. More research, however, is needed to verify this.

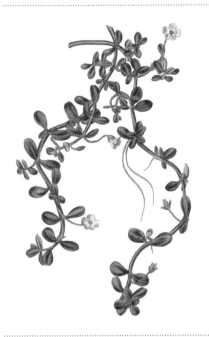

Bacopa monnieri
Bacopa, herb of grace

Creeping succulent found growing in India.

Part(s) used Aerial parts.
Traditional uses In Indian Ayurvedic medicine, herb of grace was used to improve memory and learning and to strengthen nerve function. The plant was said to help relieve pain and inflammation and to have sedative properties.
Medicinal discoveries Scientific studies have revealed that preparations of the plant and its constituents (triterpenoid saponins) might help protect nerve cells, improve memory and reduce anxiety. Clinical studies in humans showed promising effects on memory function and anxiety.

Ballota nigra
Black horehound, stinking horehound

Perennial plant with an offensive odour that is native to temperate regions of the eastern hemisphere. Produces dense whorls of lilac flowers in the autumn. Prefers alkaline soils.

Part(s) used Aerial parts.
Traditional uses It was used to treat nervous disorders, vomiting, migraine, travel sickness and sickness in the early stages of pregnancy. Sixteenth-century herbalist John Gerard (see page 81) indicated that the plant was an antidote to dog bites.
Medicinal discoveries Laboratory studies have reported sedative and anti-inflammatory properties. Clinical trials have shown that horehound decreases anxiety in patients with sleeping disorders.

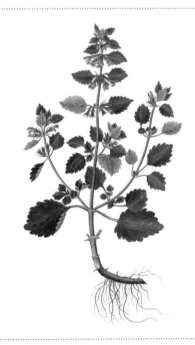

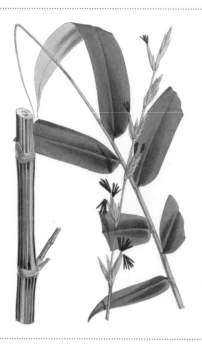

Bambusa vulgaris
Bamboo

A perennial plant, originally from Asia, with
yellow-green striped stems and dark leaves.
Suitable for many soil types, bamboo can be
grown as a feature plant, hedging or to help
stabilize areas prone to erosion.

Part(s) used Leaf, shoot and young stem.
Traditional uses Shoots were made into a
tonic to treat ulcers and wounds. Leaves were
used to treat measles, sexually transmitted
disease and various inflammatory conditions.
Medicinal discoveries Scientific studies are
being conducted on the use of young stems
in traditional Chinese medicine for coughs,
insomnia and morning sickness.

Bellis perennis
Daisy

An evergreen perennial with rosettes of
dark green, spoon-shaped leaves and small,
yellow-centred, pink-tinged white flowers.
Daisies will grow in well-drained chalk, clay,
sand or loam soils and in grass.

Part(s) used Flower.
Traditional uses It was prescribed as a
'princely remedy for old laborrs, especially
gardeners'. Used to treat joint, stomach
and liver complaints, eye problems, coughs,
colds, toothache and burns. It is used in
homeopathy for wounds and bruises
of soft tissue.
Medicinal discoveries There is research
being undertaken on the antibacterial
properties of the flowers.

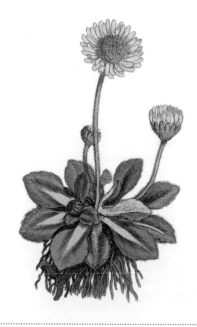

Berberis vulgaris
Barberry

Dense, thorny hedgerow shrub native to central and southern Europe with clusters of red berries and dark green foliage. There are different varieties with a range of flower colours. Grows well in most soils, except those that are waterlogged.

Part(s) used Fruit, inner bark, twig.
Traditional uses From the Middle Ages until the modern period, folk medicine was governed by the Doctrine of Signatures (see page 81). It decreed that plants which resemble various parts of the body could be used to treat those parts of the body. The yellow colour of the barberry bark was linked to the colour of people suffering from jaundice – in parts of Cornwall it was known as the 'jaundice tree'. Traditionally, the bark was cooked with stout, ale or white wine. Bark and twigs were used to treat gallstones and indigestion and to promote hair growth. An infusion of berries was taken as a tonic and to treat kidney problems. Homeopaths prescribed it for kidney and bladder problems and to help improve gallbladder function.
Medicinal discoveries Barberry contains an alkaloid compound called berberine that in laboratory and clinical studies has been shown to modulate abnormal heart rhythms. It also has antibacterial properties and can inhibit bacteria adhering to cells, which could explain why barberry is used traditionally for urinary infections.

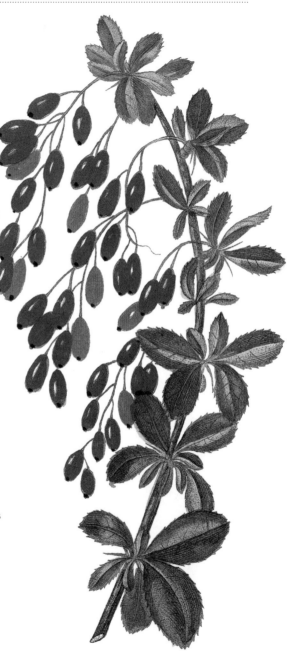

Betula pendula
Silver birch, weeping birch

Deciduous tree from northern Europe with white bark and yellow autumnal foliage.

Part(s) used Leaf.

Traditional uses Used for rheumatic complaints and gout and as a remedy for hair loss and dandruff. It was believed to be a 'spring cure' and to purify the blood. Leaf extracts were reputed to have diuretic properties and have been used in herbal medicine to treat urinary infections and inflammation of the urinary tract.

Medicinal discoveries Scientific studies revealed it may have antibacterial and diuretic effects. It has been investigated for anticancer and anti-inflammatory effects and has been of interest for use in arthritis.

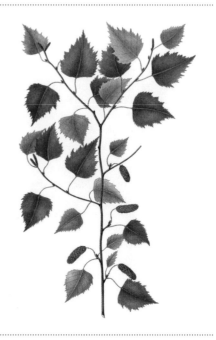

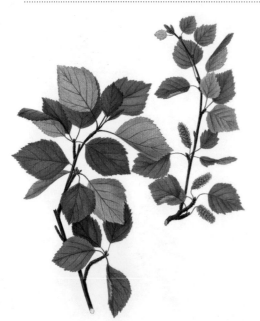

Betula pubescens
Downy birch, white birch

Native to Eurasia and introduced into N America, this deciduous tree is found growing on wet soils, such as clays and peat. It has dull grey-white bark and its flowers are produced in early spring as wind-pollinated catkins before the leaves open.

Part(s) used Bark, leaf, sap.

Traditional uses The tree sap was used to treat rheumatism, the bark to treat eczema.

Medicinal discoveries The leaves contain a compound called hyperoside that has been shown in laboratory studies to regulate the formation of urine. Clinical trials with people failed to show a significant increase in diuresis (urine production).

Borago officinalis
Starflower, borage

An annual self-seeding herb native to
the Mediterranean and Europe with
grey-green leaves and edible blue flowers.
Grows in full sun and light shade in
well-drained soils. Useful for dry places.

Part(s) used Leaf, stem, seed oil.

Traditional uses Extracts from the stems
and leaves have a wide range of traditional
uses including the treatment of gastric,
respiratory and cardiovascular disorders,
as well as coughs and fevers. Leaves were
also used to regulate hormonal systems,
including hot flushes. Herbalist John Gerard
(see page 81) reports that borage leaves
and flowers when 'put into wine make men
and women glad and merry, driving away
all sadness, dullness and melancholy'. It was
also used as a tonic for students to enable
them to concentrate.

Medicinal discoveries Borage oil has been
shown in laboratory studies and clinical
trials to alleviate stress associated with
cardiovascular conditions and to benefit
those suffering from fatigue and malaise
associated with viral infections. However,
the active components and mechanism of
action of the oil are not known, although
the oil is known to contain the fatty acid
gamma-linolenic acid which has been shown
to modulate inflammatory responses.

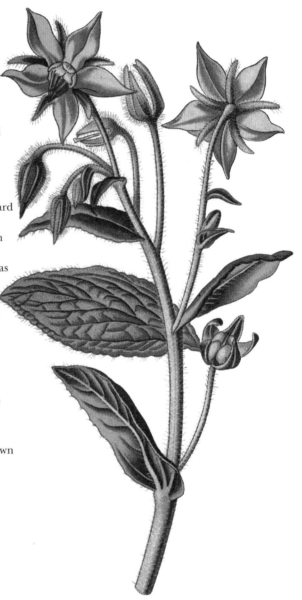

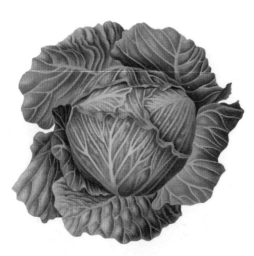

Brassica oleracea
Cabbage

Annual or biennial plants naturalized
in temperate regions. Cabbage has been
cultivated as a food plant for thousands of
years; ornamental varieties with colourful
leaves are now available.

Part(s) used Flower, leaf.
Traditional uses Leaves were used as
remedies for wounds, ulcers, eczema
and rheumatism. Herbalist John Gerard
(see page 81) reports its use for 'dim eyes,
shaking palsie' and snake bites. In folklore,
cabbages are linked to bad luck and death.
Medicinal discoveries Current interest in
cultivars of broccoli as 'superfoods' as they
contain compounds considered to have
cancer-protective properties.

Bryonia alba
White bryony

A sun-loving, herbaceous perennial vine
native to Europe and N. Iran. Its fast-
growing habit can make it invasive.

Part(s) used All parts.
Traditional uses Often confused with
mandrake because of its thick root – it was
known as the English mandrake – and
used with great caution as an aphrodisiac
and carried to ward off rheumatism.
Despite its known toxicity, roots were
used to treat hysteria, epilepsy, vertigo,
headache, migraine, melancholia, ulcers
and respiratory diseases. Homeopaths
prescribed it as a remedy for aches and pains.
Medicinal discoveries All parts of the plant
contain toxic compounds.

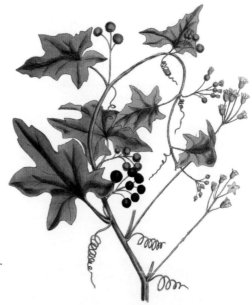

Buddleja officinalis
Butterfly bush

Native to China, this spring-flowering, deciduous shrub was first cultivated in Europe in the early nineteenth century. It has mauve to purple, fragrant, nectar-rich flowers that are highly attractive to butterflies – hence its common name, butterfly bush. It grows on poor soils, but be aware when choosing a planting site that its roots can penetrate concrete.

Part(s) used Aerial parts.

Traditional uses Extracts of the flowers were used to treat eye problems (in Chinese medicine) and burst blood vessels. Leaf and flower extracts were both used to treat gonorrhoea and hepatitis. Leaf extracts were also used to treat asthma, coughs and bronchitis.

Medicinal discoveries There is some clinical data to support the use of flower extracts as eye drops for eye diseases such as corneal glaucoma and dry eye. Evidence from laboratory studies would suggest that the flavonoid compounds in the extract modulate the activity of the tear ducts so eyes are kept moist.

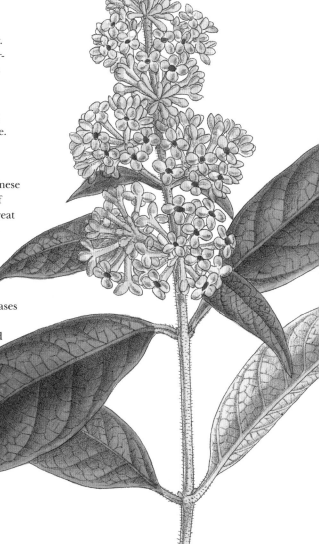

Calendula officinalis
Marigold

Nicholas Culpeper, the seventeenth-century herbalist and astrologer (see page 81), described the marigold as the 'herb of the Sun, and under Leo', probably on account of its characteristic bright orange flowers. The flowers are the parts that are usually used medicinally, although Culpeper recommends the leaves mixed with vinegar to bathe 'hot swellings'.

Marigold flowers are still widely employed across Europe for skin conditions, mostly in the form of creams and oils. They are considered beneficial for minor wounds and burns, insect bites and stings, bruises, ulcers and inflammatory skin conditions. Herbalists prescribe a tea from the flowers to heal stomach ulcers and as a gargle to soothe inflamed gums. They are also used to stimulate delayed menstruation and reduce painful periods.

Research has focused on a group of compounds called triterpenes that have proven anti-inflammatory benefits. Antibacterial and antiviral activities have also been reported. Marigold may contribute to wound healing by stimulating the growth of new blood vessels and skin tissue.

Grow An annual or biennial that grows in full sun to partial shade in well-drained soil. A native of the Mediterranean, it is now found across temperate regions. It will flower all summer until the first frost.
Harvest Pick flower heads on a dry, preferably sunny, day.

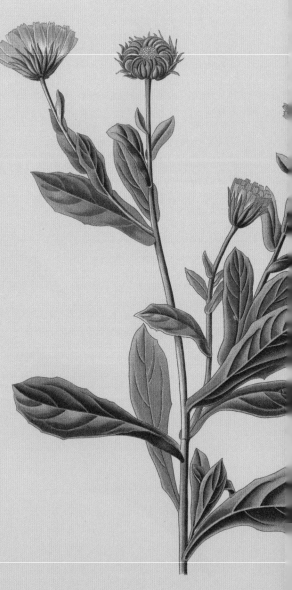

Calendula lip balm

This soothing balm harnesses calendula's healing properties to treat chapped lips and minor burns. To make the infused oil, follow the recipe on page 107 using dried calendula flowers in place of the St John's wort.

20 g (¾ oz) shea butter

20 g (¾ oz) beeswax

50 ml (2 fl oz) calendula-infused oil

15 drops lavender essential oil

You will also need: scales; heatproof bowl; large pan; oven gloves; small balm tins

1. Place the shea butter and beeswax in a heatproof bowl. Stand the bowl in a large pan of boiling water on the stove (don't let any drips of water get into the mixture) and stir occasionally until it has melted.

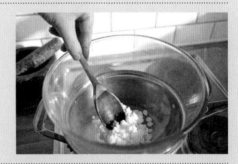

2. Wearing oven gloves, remove the bowl from the heat and stir in the calendula-infused oil and the lavender essential oil.

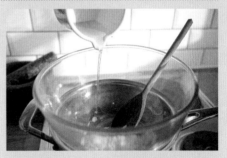

3. Carefully pour the liquid into the balm tins, filling to just below the rims. Leave to cool, then pop on the lids. Will keep for one year.

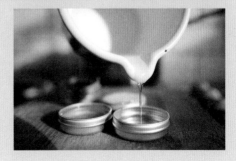

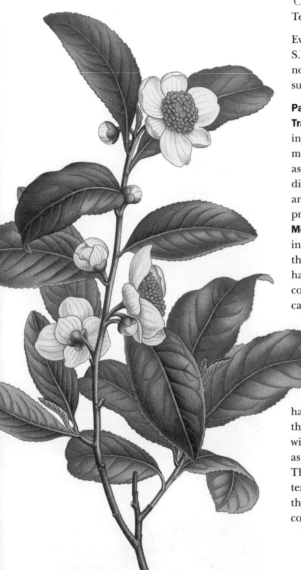

Camellia sinensis
Tea

Evergreen shrub that is native to E. and
S.E. Asia and the Indian subcontinent,
now grown worldwide in the tropics and
subtropics.

Part(s) used Leaf.

Traditional uses The leaves have been used
in traditional Chinese medicine and other
medical systems such as Ayurveda to treat
asthma as well as vascular and coronary
diseases. In China, spring-harvested leaves
are thought to have the best health-giving
properties.

Medicinal discoveries There is increased
interest in the compounds called catechins
that occur in tea leaves. These compounds
have anti-inflammatory activity and could
contribute to why tea has been used to treat
cardiovascular diseases. These compounds
can play a role in the regulation of
glucose in the blood and there
is increased interest in the use
of these compounds to further
our knowledge about Type 2
diabetes. Results of clinical trials
have also indicated that tea might delay
the onset of some symptoms associated
with neurodegenerative conditions such
as Alzheimer's or Parkinson's disease.
The majority of the health benefits of
tea are associated with green tea, not
the fermented black tea that is mostly
consumed in the West.

Cannabis sativa
Cannabis, marijuana

Generally grows as an annual and is thought to have originated from Central Asia. It is a short-day plant and only starts flowering in late summer when the day length starts to shorten. The plant has characteristic digitate serrate leaflets. In many parts of the world it is illegal to grow the plant without having an appropriate licence.

Part(s) used Flower buds, resin.
Traditional uses Records show that cannabis was traditionally used initially by the Chinese for its mind-altering properties and then taken into the Middle East by the early Scythians, thence to Europe and Africa and from Africa into South America and North America. It was used in Asia as an anesthetic during surgery, to stimulate the appetite and as a tonic.
Medicinal discoveries Cannabinoids are considered to be the key compounds associated with the medicinal uses of cannabis. These compounds are being tested as single compounds or as simple mixtures, not as crude plant extracts. Many clinical trials are currently taking place to evaluate their use for the treatment of pain and other symptoms associated with multiple sclerosis, rheumatoid arthritis and for the control of cancer pain that is not responding to morphine.

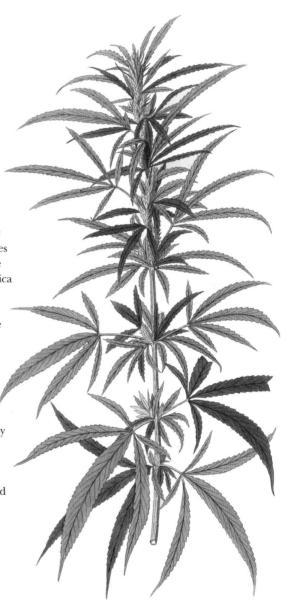

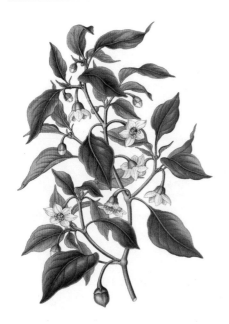

Capsicum annuum
Chilli

Originally from S. America, this shrub will grow in most climates. Grows well in pots, but don't let the compost get either too wet or dry or it will drop its leaves. The fruits, known as peppers, can vary in colour from yellow-green to dark red-black. Flowers are small and white, tinged with purple.

Part(s) used Fruit, leaf.
Traditional uses Leaves were used to cure toothache. The fruit was used to stimulate gastric juices and treat gastric disorders, chronic laryngitis, chilblains and rheumatism. It was given to women suffering pain during childbirth.
Medicinal discoveries Products containing capsaicin are used to relieve osteoarthritis.

Carex arenaria
Sand sedge

Perennial that occurs along sandy coasts in Britain and Europe. Planted in sand dunes to help stabilize them. Some *Carex* species are grown as ornamentals.

Part(s) used Root.
Traditional uses In parts of Europe, the roots were considered to have diuretic properties and to increase sweating.
Medicinal discoveries The sand sedge has not been widely studied for its medicinal properties. *Carex folliculata* and *C. gynandra* have been explored for their potential anticancer effects.

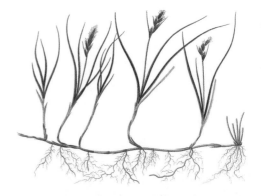

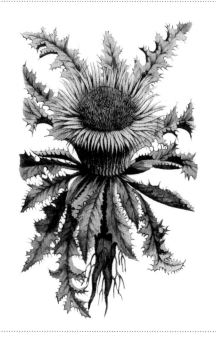

Carlina acaulis
Carline thistle

Perennial or biennial with spiny leaves and disc-shaped flowers that occurs in grassland and mountainous areas in Europe.

Part(s) used Root.
Traditional uses In medieval times, the roots were considered an antidote to poison. Believed to have diuretic properties, and used for liver problems. Also reputed to alleviate skin eruptions and used as a wash for wounds and ulcers.
Medicinal discoveries Some scientific studies suggest the carline thistle has antimicrobial and antitrypanosomal effects. It has not been explored scientifically as extensively as other thistles, such as milk thistle (*Silybum marianum*).

Carthamus tinctorius
Safflower, saffron thistle

An annual of the daisy family (Asteraceae) with spiny leaves and yellow or orange flowers.

Part(s) used Flower, seed.
Traditional uses Used for measles, other skin eruptions and fevers, and to stimulate the heart and circulation. Used in traditional Chinese medicine to promote menstruation. Flowers were reputed as laxative and to promote sweating.
Medicinal discoveries Safflower preparations have been investigated for effects on blood pressure, the immune system, for anti-inflammatory and anticoagulant activities, and for potential to protect nerve cells. Seed oil has been used in some nutritional regimens.

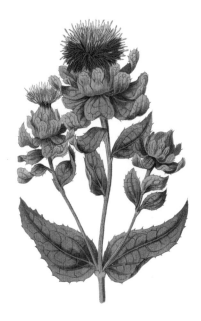

Carum carvi
Caraway

Biennial herb cultivated in Europe,
N. Africa and Australia with finely divided,
feathery leaves. Leaves and seeds have an
aniseed-liquorice taste.

Part(s) used Seed.
Traditional uses Long-established treatment
for digestive disorders, bloating, loss of
appetite and in tonics to decrease phlegm,
relieve constipation and menstrual cramps,
and to freshen the breath.
Medicinal discoveries In clinical studies it
has been shown to decrease pain in patients
with digestive disorders. It has carminative
(combats flatulence) and antibacterial
activity. It is added to mouthwashes,
toothpaste and cosmetics.

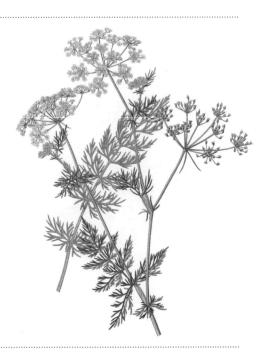

Castanea sativa
Sweet chestnut

Long-lived, widely cultivated, deciduous
woodland tree from N. Africa and
S. Europe. The flowers appear after the
leaves in summer; in autumn the female
flowers develop into spiny nuts.

Part(s) used Fruit, leaf.
Traditional uses Leaves were used to make
a tonic and to treat fevers, dysentery,
diarrhoea, coughs, especially whooping
cough, and wounds including mouth sores.
Used in homeopathy for anxiety.
Medicinal discoveries Scientific studies
have shown fruit and leaf extracts have
antibacterial and antioxidant activity.

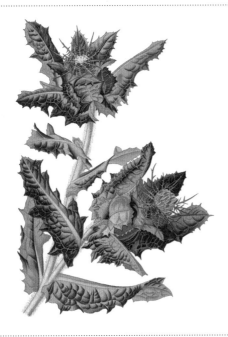

Centaurea benedicta

Holy thistle, blessed thistle

Annual thistle, native to S. Europe.

Part(s) used Aerial parts.
Traditional uses Reputed to purify and aid blood circulation and strengthen the brain and memory. The sixteenth-century botanist William Turner claimed it was 'good for the headache', 'for any ache in the body', and that 'there is nothing better for the canker and old rotten and festering sores than the leaves, juice, broth, powder and water' of the holy thistle. It was a reputed plague cure. Also used as a bitter to stimulate appetite and in homeopathic medicines.
Medicinal discoveries Extracts of the plant have antimicrobial properties and might have potential to protect nerve cells.

Centaurium erythraea

Centaury

Small biennial native to dry grasslands in Europe and W. Asia. Produces pink flowers.

Part(s) used Aerial parts.
Traditional uses In Greek mythology, the centaur Chiron cured a wound from a poison arrow with centaury. Culpeper describes how preparations 'dropped into the ears cleanseth them from worms, foul ulcers and spreading scabs of the head'. Centaury was a remedy for appetite loss, kidney and bladder disorders and for clearing 'the eyes of dimness and clouds'.
Medicinal discoveries Scientific studies suggest centaury has anti-inflammatory and fever-reducing effects. It is undergoing tests for its anti-ulcer and sedative properties.

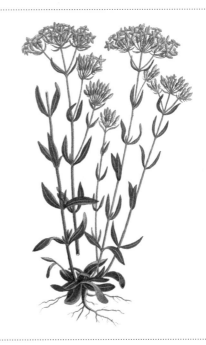

Centella asiatica
Gotu kola

Creeping perennial from Asia and Australia that produces kidney-shaped leaves and small pink-red flowers. Spreads rapidly.

Part(s) used Aerial parts.

Traditional uses Used as a diuretic and antirheumatic and to heal wounds, ulcers and other skin complaints. In Ayurvedic medicine, gotu kola was reputed to prevent dementia and promote longevity. It was used in India and Africa to treat leprosy. In traditional Chinese medicine it was used to combat physical and mental exhaustion.

Medicinal discoveries Scientific studies have revealed that preparations of the plant and its constituents (triterpenoids) might protect and repair damaged nerve cells. Some preliminary clinical trials in humans suggest that gotu kola might improve memory and reduce stress and anxiety. Laboratory studies also revealed that the triterpenoids have wound-healing and anti-inflammatory properties. Thus, gotu kola preparations have been investigated for their potential to aid wound-healing, reduce scar formation and alleviate psoriasis.

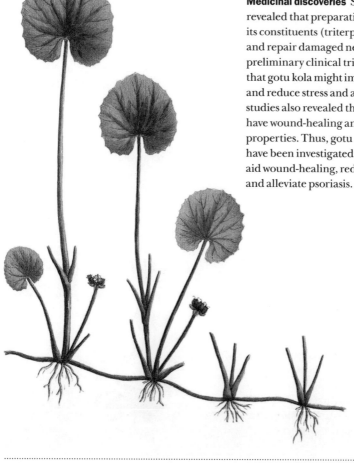

Chaenomeles sinensis
Chinese quince

Deciduous shrub native to Asia, with spiny twigs. Produces white, pink or red spring flowers, depending on the cultivar.

Part(s) used Fruit.
Traditional uses A traditional Chinese medicine known for centuries as a remedy for inflammation and spasms, and as a stimulant for digestion and circulation.
Medicinal discoveries Fruit preparations have been investigated for their antiviral effects against influenza, their anticancer activity and for their potential to aid memory. Fruit constituents have shown some effects on nerve growth in laboratory studies.

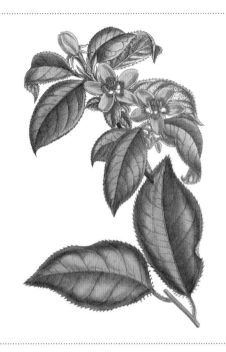

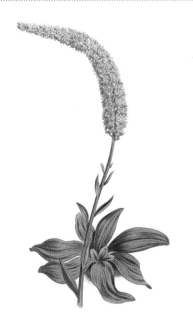

Chamaelirium luteum
Blazing star, false unicorn

N. American herbaceous perennial with white flowers. Grows in shaded areas and woodland gardens.

Part(s) used Root.
Traditional uses Reputed to alleviate depression and 'derangements of women'. Considered a remedy for menstrual disorders, menopausal symptoms, infertility and intestinal worms. Used traditionally by Native North Americans to prevent miscarriage.
Medicinal discoveries In preliminary scientific studies, when combined with other herbal medicines, the roots of false unicorn show antitumor activity, while steroidal type compounds from the root also have anticancer effects.

Chamaemelum nobile
Roman chamomile

Roman chamomile flowers are taken as a tea for a wide range of digestive ills including diarrhoea, acid reflux, travel sickness, spasm, wind and indigestion. In studies they have been shown to have antispasmodic and anti-inflammatory actions. The tea has a sedative effect, improves sleep and reduces feelings of anxiety.

Maud Grieve, an early twentieth-century gardener and herbalist, described it as 'wonderfully soothing and sedative' and 'the sole certain remedy for nightmare'. It is considered by some as the 'plant's physician' for its reputed restorative effect on other plants. It is often grown as an ornamental scented lawn. In ancient Greek, chamomile means 'ground apple', after its habitat and scent when crushed.

Chamomile flower preparations are used externally as an emollient (to retain moisture) and as an anti-inflammatory for dry, inflamed skin conditions such as eczema. It is an ingredient in cosmetics and hair-lightening products. Rub used chamomile tea bags over the skin as a cleanser and to soothe inflammation.

Grow Native to W. Europe. Prefers well-drained soil in sun or partial shade. Mat-forming, chamomile can spread to 50 cm (20 in). Flowers through summer.
Harvest Pick flowers by combing your fingers through the plant.
Caution May cause allergic reactions, such as dermatitis, if sensitive to plants of the daisy (Asteraceae) family.

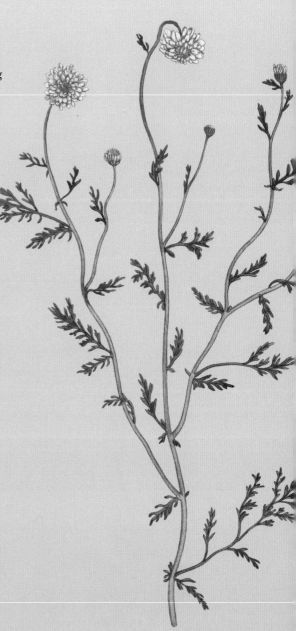

Chamomile cream

This recipe for a cooling moisturiser uses an extract of chamomile flowers. The addition of lavender essential oil augments the cream's calming and anti-inflammatory properties.

30 g (1 oz) dried chamomile flowers

   or 100 g (3½ oz) fresh chamomile flowers

200 ml (7 fl oz) boiling water

100 g (3½ oz) base cream

20 drops lavender essential oil

You will also need: scales; cafetière; measuring jug;

   glass bowl; spatula; sterilized, airtight jars

1. Place flowers in a cafetière (ensure the glass and plunger are clean and free of any traces of coffee) and pour over boiling water. Cover and leave to cool. Press down the plunger and pour out 30 ml (1 fl oz) of tea.

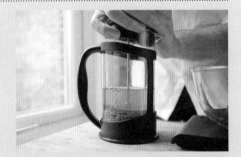

2. Spoon the base cream into a clean bowl. Trickle over the tea, a few teaspoonfuls at a time, stirring vigorously until it's completely mixed in. Then stir in twenty drops of lavender essential oil. The consistency should be thick and creamy.

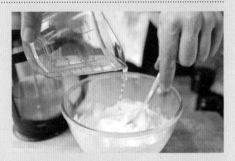

3. Using a spatula or butter knife, transfer the cream into small, sterilized, air-tight jars. Store cream in the fridge and use within three months.

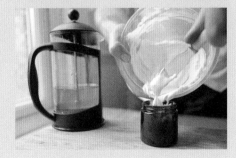

Chelidonium majus
Greater celandine

A perennial plant that will grow in most soils, it produces yellow flowers from spring to summer. If not controlled it can be an invasive weed.

Part(s) used Aerial parts, sap.
Traditional uses It was taken as a mild analgesic and sedative and to treat blood disorders, gallstones and bacterial infections. The latex-like sap was used to seal open wounds, as a tonic to purify the blood and applied topically to corns and warts.
Medicinal discoveries Research has shown that the plant contains toxic alkaloids, such as coptisine, so should be prescribed only by a professional herbalist or pharmacist.

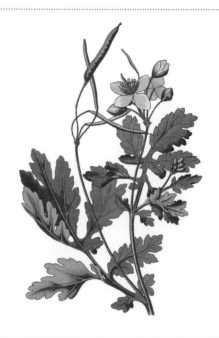

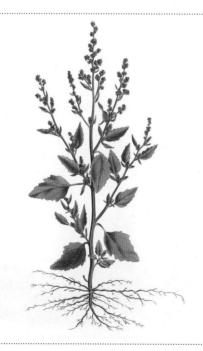

Chenopodium album
Fat hen

Annual with grey-green leaves and flowers that bloom from summer to autumn. Grows on most soils and is considered a weed. The seeds were fed to poultry to fatten them, hence its common name.

Part(s) used Aerial parts.
Traditional uses Extracts from aerial parts were used to treat rheumatism and gout and as a mild laxative. Leaves were applied as a wash or poultice to insect bites and sunstroke and as a decoction to treat toothache. Seeds were chewed to treat urinary problems.
Medicinal discoveries There is some evidence that when the aerial parts are added to food, fat hen can aid those suffering from anaemia.

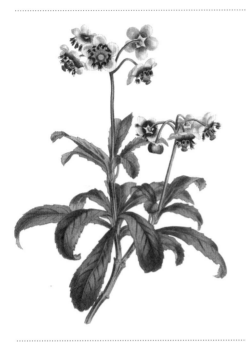

Chimaphila umbellata
Western prince's pine, pipsissewa

Evergreen perennial shrub from cool regions of Eurasia and N. America. Produces clusters of pink-white flowers.

Part(s) used Whole plant.
Traditional uses It was considered a remedy for bladder problems and was used as a diuretic tonic for the kidneys and spleen. Used by Native North Americans for rheumatic complaints.
Medicinal discoveries Preparations have shown anti-inflammatory and antioxidant effects. Scientific studies also revealed preparations have antifungal and antibacterial properties. It is being investigated for effects on prostate disorders.

Chrysanthemum indicum
Indian chrysanthemum, Japanese chrysanthemum

Perennial native to China. Its foliage has a pungent but refreshing, lemon-like fragrance. Will grow in most soils in full sun.

Part(s) used Aerial parts.
Traditional uses Wide range of traditional uses as blood tonic, to treat eye ailments, hypertension, respiratory diseases, migraine, boils and eczema. Used in traditional Chinese medicine to treat inflammation, hypertension and respiratory diseases.
Medicinal discoveries The essential oil contains chrysanthenone, which is being studied for its action on parts of the brain affected by Parkinson's disease.

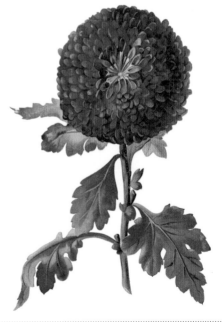

Cichorium intybus
Chicory

Although some people may consider it a weed, chicory's stunning, bright blue flowers make an attractive addition to a herbaceous border. The plant's bitter flavour acts to stimulate the appetite and improve digestion. In southern Europe the leaves are commonly gathered from the wild and eaten at the start of a meal, simply fried in oil and garlic or enjoyed in a salad.

Chicory shares many of its traditional uses with its cousin, the dandelion: it is recommended for poor appetite, general stomach ache, gallstones, as a mild laxative and as a general tonic for the liver. Its use in the treatment of digestive dysfunction can be explained in part by the high inulin content of the root (around 50 per cent). Inulin is a carbohydrate that is not broken down by the human digestive system; it survives intact into the lower gut where 'good' bacteria feed off it. Inulin also has a mild laxative effect.

Grow Grows in most soils, found wild in the UK in lime-rich areas. Can grow to height of 2 m (6½ ft) and spreads to 50 cm (20 in).
Harvest Dig up roots after the plant has finished flowering in the autumn.

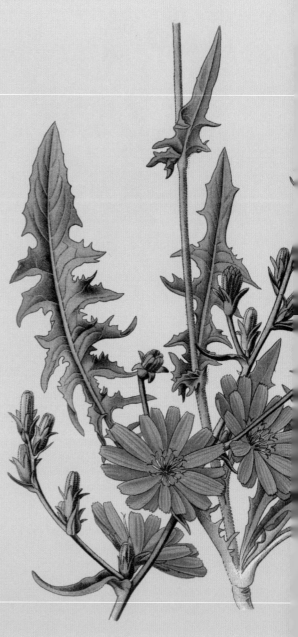

Chicory coffee

Making chicory coffee is simple and the roasting roots are wonderfully aromatic. Drink one to two cups a day to support bowel flora after an infection, antibiotics, stress or a poor or changed diet. Add up to two teaspoonfuls of the ground roasted chicory to a cafetière, pour on hot water and brew for five minutes.

Large handful of chicory roots

You will also need: knife; baking tray; spice grinder; sterilized airtight jar with lid

1. Scrub roots in water with a stiff brush to remove any mud. Pat dry with a tea towel or kitchen paper.

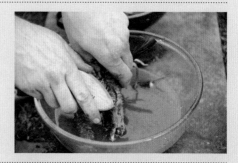

2. Finely slice the roots into rounds.

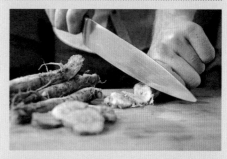

3. Spread the pieces evenly across a baking tray in a single layer. Put in an oven preheated to 180°C/350°F for two hours, checking occasionally that the chicory isn't burning – turn the oven down if this is the case. Turn the oven off and leave to cool. Store in an airtight jar and grind the chicory as and when you want it.

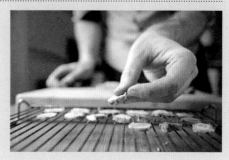

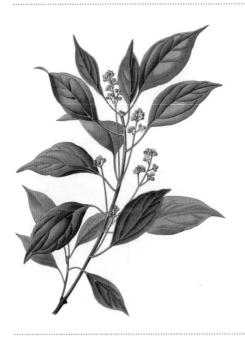

Cinnamomum camphora
Camphor laurel, camphor tree

Evergreen tree with shiny aromatic leaves and clusters of cream flowers. Occurs in China and Japan.

Part(s) used Wood.
Traditional uses Camphor extracted from the wood was thought to calm nervousness and hysteria. It was also used to combat chills, colds and inflammatory conditions, and to treat fevers and pneumonia. Preparations were applied to sprains and rheumatic complaints.
Medicinal discoveries Camphor is used in ointments and liniments to alleviate aches and pains. It is an ingredient in some inhaled decongestant preparations for cold and flu symptoms. May have an irritant effect.

Cirsium heterophyllum
Melancholy thistle

Perennial thistle that occurs in Scotland and other parts of Britain. Other species are more often grown as ornamentals, such as the Japanese thistle (*Cirsium japonicum*).

Part(s) used Leaf, root.
Traditional uses In the seventeenth century, melancholy thistle wine was drunk to 'expel superfluous melancholy out of the body and makes a man as merry as a cricket'. In Asia, the Japanese thistle was used to treat bleeding disorders.
Medicinal discoveries The melancholy thistle has not yet been assessed for its medicinal properties. However, the Japanese thistle has been investigated for anti-anxiety and antidepressant effects.

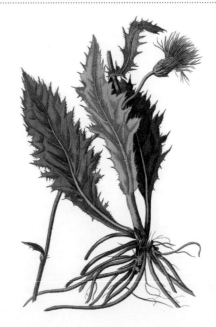

Citrullus colocynthis
Bitter apple, colocynth

Native to N. Africa and W. Asia, this perennial vine produces small yellow and green striped gourds.

Part(s) used Fruit.
Traditional uses Bitter apple is considered to be the wild gourd described in the Bible. The fruit pulp was traditionally taken as a laxative but this use fell into decline due to its aggressive purgative properties that could cause violent griping, pain and even death. It was used traditionally in parts of Asia for diabetes.
Medicinal discoveries There has been some interest in its antidiabetic effects.

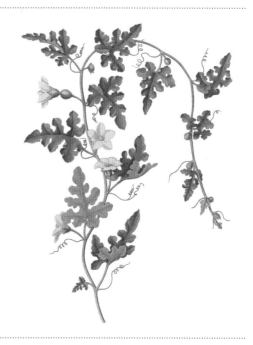

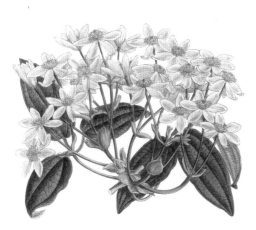

Clematis armandii
Clematis

Native to China and introduced into England in the 1900s, this vigorous climber has long, mid-green leaves and fragrant white flowers that appear in early spring. Best grown against a sheltered wall protected from cold winds.

Part(s) used Leaf, stem.
Traditional uses Used to treat cancerous and foul-smelling ulcers as well as infections such as syphilis. In traditional Chinese medicine, the stems (Chuan Mu Tong) are given for urinary and skin problems.
Medicinal discoveries Scientific evidence suggests that it has anti-inflammatory properties that could explain its use for eczema and urinary infections.

Coix lacryma-jobi
Job's tears

Annual grass that occurs in S.E. Asia and has been cultivated as an ornamental for centuries. Female flowers occur in a green, tear-shaped husk that turns grey.

Part(s) used Seed.
Traditional uses The seed has been used in traditional Chinese medicine to relieve pain, inflammation and spasms. Reputed to have antidiarrhoeal, antirheumatic and diuretic properties. Also used as a tonic for the spleen, to lower fevers and fight infections. In parts of S. America, the fruits were worn as a necklace to prevent tooth decay.
Medicinal discoveries Seeds are of interest for potential anticancer properties.

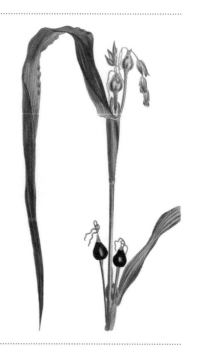

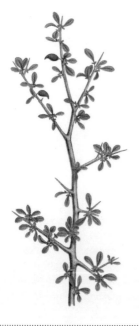

Commiphora myrrha
Myrrh

Small, bushy tree with sharp spines found in hot, rocky areas of the Middle East. Needs a warm, sheltered spot – ideally a conservatory or greenhouse. Makes a good bonsai tree.

Part(s) used Bark resin.
Traditional uses Myrrh oil was used for ulcers, indigestion, respiratory problems, arthritis, cancer, leprosy and syphilis. The Ancient Egyptians used it to delay ageing, maintain healthy skin and in embalming. In Ayurvedic and Chinese medicines it was used to treat arthritis and rheumatism.
Medicinal discoveries Scientific studies have supported the anti-inflammatory properties of the oil. Myrrh is used in aromatherapy and cosmetics.

Convallaria majalis
Lily of the valley

A rhizomatous perennial native to cool temperate areas in the northern hemisphere and Asia. It has small, fragrant, bell-shaped, white flowers with red fruits. Needs a humus-rich moist soil out of direct sun; ideal for planting under roses and shrubs. It is the national flower of Finland.

Part(s) used Flowering aerial parts.
Traditional uses Despite being highly toxic, lily of the valley has a long history of being used as a tonic for heart and gastric problems and for its anti-arrhythmic, hypertensive, diuretic and antispasmodic activities. Currently used by herbalists in Europe as a restricted herbal remedy to strengthen heart functions in patients with mild heart conditions.

Medicinal discoveries The traditional medicinal properties can be partly explained by the range of compounds known as cardiac glycosides that occur in most parts of the plant. It has similar – but milder – effects on the heart compared to those observed with *Digitalis*. However, there is less scientific data to support the use of lily of the valley compared to the extensive literature on *Digitalis*.

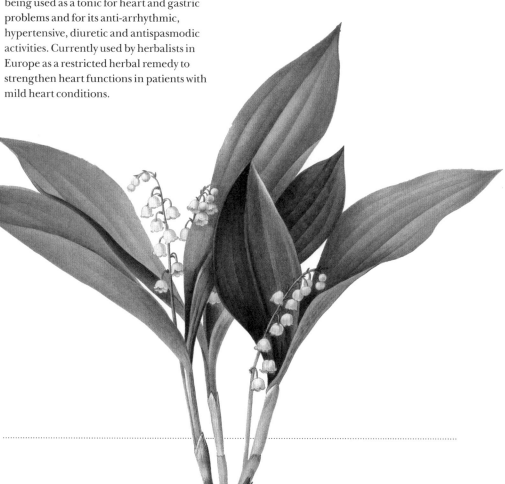

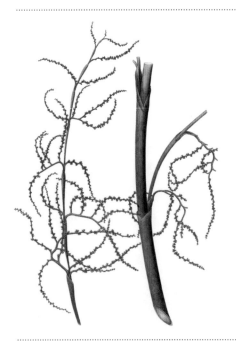

Copernicia prunifera
Carnauba wax palm

Attractive, tall-growing palm that is native to
S. America. The waxy secretion on its leaves is
harvested as a valuable commercial crop.

Part(s) used Leaf.
Traditional uses Used in Brazil and other
parts of the Americas for the reputed
laxative properties. It was also used as
a remedy for rheumatic pain. A tea was
prepared from the leaves to purify the blood.
Medicinal discoveries The carnauba wax is
used as a coating agent in pharmaceutical
formulations such as tablets. The wax is also
permitted for use in some foods and it is
used in the manufacture of some polishes
and candles.

Coriandrum sativum
Coriander, cilantro

Annual native to S. Europe, N. Africa and
S.W. Asia with small white-pink flowers. Now
grown worldwide as a culinary herb for its
leaves and seeds. Plant in a sunny spot in
well-drained, loamy soil.

Part(s) used Leaf, seed.
Traditional uses Wide range of uses including
the treatment of diabetes, blood pressure,
ulcers, urinary tract infections, anxiety,
skin problems and liver diseases. Used in
Ayurvedic medicine for treating diabetes,
kidney problems and brain function.
Medicinal discoveries Laboratory studies
have shown that as well as having anti-
inflammatory activity, it can increase insulin
release and relieve flatulence.

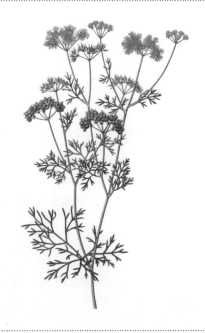

Growing medicinal plants

When choosing which plants to grow in your garden, especially long-lived trees and shrubs, remember this simple mantra: right plant, right place. Do your research, find out about a plant's life cycle, when it can be planted, how it is pollinated and when it should be pruned. Consider the habitat you can offer in your garden and compare it to where the plant is found growing in the wild. You need to be able to match the site (for example, sun, shade, partial shade, sheltered), soil type (acid, alkaline, neutral) and growing conditions (rocky outcrops, boggy ground or grassland). Be wary of fast-growing plants with lush vegetation as they may take over your garden.

The temperature range the plant can cope with is key, too. Many species used to a warmer, semi-tropical climate can be grown in more temperate conditions if you keep them protected from winter frosts, cold winds and persistent wet. It's also worth asking a good plant supplier if a hardier variety has been bred.

Growing and propagating plants is hugely rewarding – even more so if the plants are culturally or medically important. But simply providing the right growing environment doesn't always guarantee success. The medicinal properties of plants are known to be influenced by a wide range of environmental factors, such as soil conditions, sunlight and water. The chemically active properties also vary among individual plants. One of the most famous examples of this relates to the South American cinchona tree. The active compound in its bark is quinine, which was used to treat malaria. Back in the 1800s many trips were made to South America to collect cinchona seedlings which were taken to different parts of Asia. As the trees matured their bark was harvested but found not to contain quinine. Further collections were made from plants known to contain quinine and plantations were often created using vegetatively propagated trees.

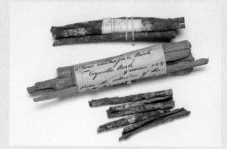

Cinchona **bark specimens.**

Crataegus monogyna
Common hawthorn

Now renowned for use in heart conditions, references of the middle ages focus on its use in nervous conditions. This is still linked to the art as anxiety can produce over stimulation of the 'fight or flight response' causing an increase in heart rate. Hawthorn is well studied, and has been shown to increase the force of contraction of the heart, whilst slowing the rate. There is also evidence that it improves circulation to the tissues of the heart and reduces cardiovascular disease risk. It is used as a traditional remedy for high blood pressure, heart arrhythmia, angina and Raynaud's disease.

Hawthorn has been grown for thousands of years as a dense hedge to deter humans and animals. It was important in pagan fertility rituals, as the blossoms marked the arrival of spring. The young leaves can be eaten as a salad. The red berries brighten an otherwise dull looking late autumn garden.

Grow This hardy hedgerow tree will cope with most planting sites and soils. Spring flowers are followed by berries that ripen to red in autumn.
Harvest Pick leaves and flowers together in spring. Wait until the berries have reddened and the leaves have dropped before picking.
Safety Check with a health professional before taking hawthorn preparations if you have any cardiovascular conditions.

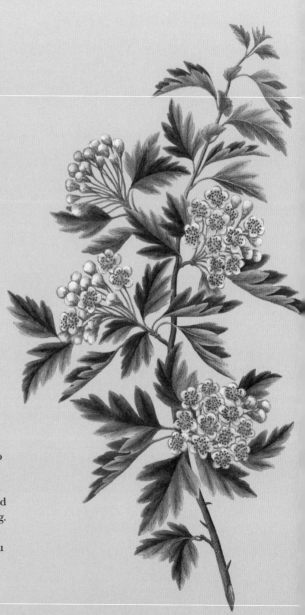

Hawthorn spiced wine

Before distilling was invented, infused wines were a common way of taking medicine. As well as hawthorn, this recipe includes other herbs considered to improve circulation and have warming properties. Take 5 ml (1 teaspoon) twice a day, or drink one small sherry glassful daily, to support general circulation.

5 cm (2 in) piece fresh ginger

2 tablespoons muscovado sugar

2 cinnamon sticks

40–50 fresh hawthorn berries

250 ml (9 fl oz) red wine

You will also need: sharp knife; pestle and mortar; measuring jug; muslin; funnel; sterilized lidded jar; bottle with stopper

1. Peel and dice the ginger and place in the jar with the sugar. Grind the cinnamon sticks in a pestle and mortar or spice grinder and add to the jar.

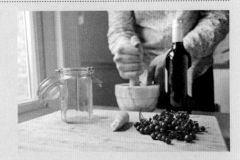

2. Add the hawthorn berries to the jar and press down with a spoon to crush them. Pour over the wine and mix well.

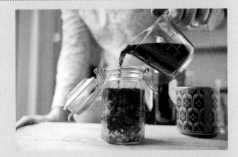

3. Leave the mixture in a cool, dark place, turning the jar every day. If the level of wine drops, add more to keep the berries covered. After one week, strain the liquid through a funnel lined with muslin into a sterilized bottle. The wine will keep for up to six weeks.

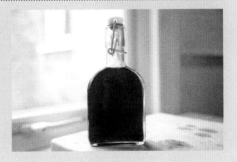

Crithmum maritimum
Rock samphire

Salt-tolerant perennial found along the coastlines of S. and W. Britain, Ireland and the Mediterranean. A good plant for a rock garden, it grows readily in most free-draining soils. Fleshy, blue-green stems and leaves with yellow-green summer flowers.

Part(s) used Leaf.
Traditional uses Leaf extracts used as a diuretic and as a remedy for scurvy and digestive and kidney problems. Young leaves were consumed to relieve flatulence and promote weight loss.
Medicinal discoveries The essential oil from the leaves has antibacterial properties. Leaves contain vitamin C which could explain why it was eaten to treat scurvy.

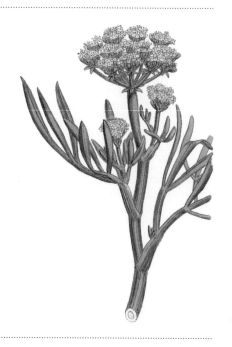

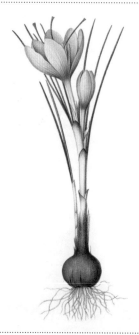

Crocus sativus
Saffron

Plant autumn-flowering saffron bulbs in the border or a container to enjoy their vibrant purple flowers and orange stamens. Give them a sunny spot in gritty, well-drained soil or compost. Avoid overwatering.

Part(s) used Flower stamen.
Traditional uses Used to treat stomach problems, gum pains and coughs. As a tonic it was reported to have sedative properties.
Medicinal discoveries The flower stamens contain the compound crocin, which has antidepressant properties. Saffron has also been investigated for pain relief and for treating anxiety in patients with Alzheimer's disease.

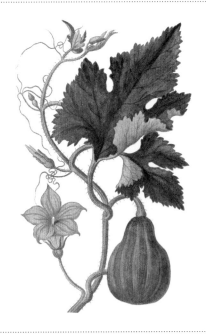

Cucurbita pepo
Squash, pumpkin

This annual vine is thought to be one of the oldest domesticated species from S. America. There are many different cultivars with various coloured fruits. Grow in warm conditions and keep well watered when flowering and fruiting.

Part(s) used Fruit, leaf, sap, seed.
Traditional uses In C. and N. America, sap was applied to burns, seeds were used as a diuretic, for de-worming and for treating bronchitis and fever. In Ayurvedic medicine, fruits were used to purify the blood and leaves used as a painkiller and to treat nausea.
Medicinal discoveries Laboratory studies have shown that leaves have antiviral and anti-inflammatory activity.

Cuminum cyminum
Cumin

Thought to be native to Egypt, annual cumin tolerates a wide range of soil types, but will do best in well-drained, fertile soil in full sun. It is drought-tolerant and requires a long growing season to produce seeds. Has white or pink flowers.

Part(s) used Seed.
Traditional uses In Sanskrit cumin was known as *jira*, 'that which helps digestion'. It was used to treat heart disease, swellings, vomiting and chronic fever.
Medicinal discoveries There is current interest in developing the compounds isolated from the seeds for their cancer-protective properties and as a drug for use in treating angina and asthma.

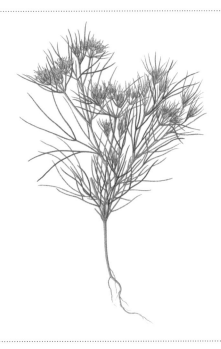

Curcuma longa
Turmeric

Perennial with yellow-white and pink flowers. It occurs in parts of Asia and species also grow in Australia.

Part(s) used Rhizome.

Traditional uses Turmeric has been used in traditional Ayurvedic and Chinese medicines to aid digestion and to counteract liver disorders. It was also used for its reputed diuretic properties, and as a remedy for rheumatic complaints and menstrual disorders. It was applied to the skin to treat ulcers, scabies, wounds and eczema. In Ayurvedic medicine, turmeric was regarded as a rejuvenator to slow the ageing process. According to the Pharmacopoeia of the People's Republic of China, it was a remedy for mania.

Medicinal discoveries Scientific studies have revealed that turmeric has many biological activities, including antitumour, anti-inflammatory and anti-ulcer effects. Studies also suggest it may help protect the liver, heal wounds and reduce cholesterol. Clinical trials in humans appear to support some of these uses, although more robust studies are needed. There has been much interest in the potential anticancer, cholesterol-lowering and anti-inflammatory properties of turmeric. Studies also suggest that populations that consume curry which contains turmeric might have a lower risk of dementia, so it has been investigated for potential benefits in Alzheimer's disease. Also a source of yellow and orange dyes.

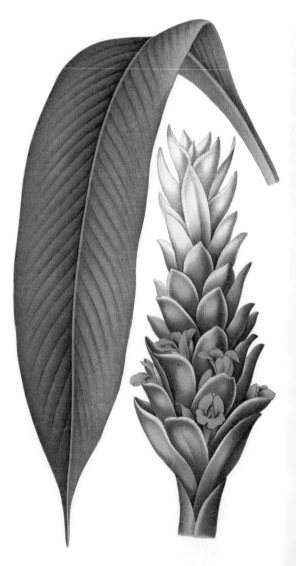

Cucumis sativus

Cucumber

Trailing annual, native to India. Produces yellow funnel-shaped flowers followed by elongated fruits.

Part(s) used Fruit, seed.
Traditional uses Cucumber seeds were used as a diuretic, and for catarrh, bowel and urinary problems. The leaves, stems and roots were used in traditional Chinese medicine as antidiarrhoeal and detoxifying remedies.
Medicinal discoveries Scientific studies suggest cucumber has antioxidant, antidiabetic and cholesterol-lowering properties. Seeds have been investigated for their potential to protect against ulcers. Cucumber is also used in cosmetics.

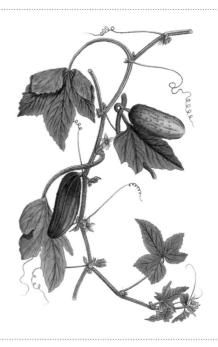

Cyamopsis tetragonoloba

Guar bean, cluster bean

Mainly cultivated in India as a fodder crop, but also grown in some regions of the Americas and Australia.

Part(s) used Seed (endosperm).
Traditional uses Mainly used as a food source, although in India it was given as a laxative and as a treatment for gastric ulcers and diabetes.
Medicinal discoveries Guar gum is used in the control of diabetes as it reduces blood sugar levels and can affect gastric emptying (how fast food leaves the stomach). It is also used to control high cholesterol. Its thickening properties are employed in the formulations of tablets and suspensions.

Cydonia oblonga
Quince

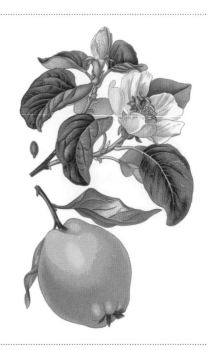

Deciduous, bush-like tree from S.W. Asia. Quince is resistant to frost and requires a cold period below 7°C/45°F to produce white-pink flowers. Edible fruits resemble a small pear and are golden-yellow when mature.

Part(s) used Fruit, leaf, seed.
Traditional uses The fruit was given for diarrhoea, cardiovascular diseases and to soothe stomach aches. The leaves were used to treat diabetes. The seeds soaked in water produce a gel that was applied to chapped lips and mouth ulcers.
Medicinal discoveries The plant is currently undergoing evaluation as a treatment for cardiovascular diseases and diabetes.

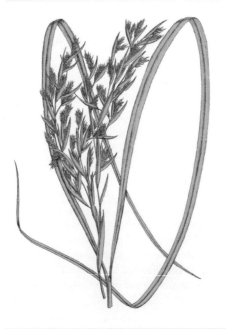

Cymbopogon citratus
Lemon grass

Rapid-growing, tropical grass from S. Asia with aromatic leaves. Makes a pretty ornamental for containers or the herb garden. Grows in most soils in sun.

Part(s) used Leaf.
Traditional uses Leaves reported to have hypnotic, anticatarrhal and anticonvulsant properties. The essential oil was used as an antiflatulent, analgesic and antimicrobial agent as well as reducing fevers. Still used in herbal and homeopathic remedies.
Medicinal discoveries Laboratory studies have shown that compounds in the essential oils from the leaves, such as citronellal and geraniol, could explain some of the traditional uses.

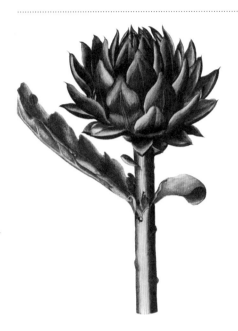

Cynara cardunculus
Cardoon

Statuesque, thistle-like, herbaceous perennial with grey-hairy, lobed leaves and rounded purple flowerheads in late summer. Ornamental varieties are available.

Part(s) used Leaf (before flowering).
Traditional uses Leaves traditionally used to treat liver, gall-bladder problems, hepatitis, arteriosclerosis and diabetes. Leaf extracts were used in herbal medicine for digestive and urinary problems.
Medicinal discoveries Cynarin, a compound isolated from the leaves, stimulates the secretion of digestive juices, in particular bile. Clinical trials have shown it lowers blood lipids.

Daphne genkwa
Daphne

A slow-growing, evergreen, woodland shrub native to China. Fragrant purple flowers appear in late winter to early spring. Dwarf cultivars are suitable for rock gardens.

Part(s) used Flower bud.
Traditional uses This toxic plant was considered one of the fifty fundamental herbs in traditional Chinese medicine. It was prescribed for a diverse range of ailments including arthritis, and for pain relief.
Medicinal discoveries There is current interest in the anticancer activity of the diterpenoid compounds isolated from this plant.

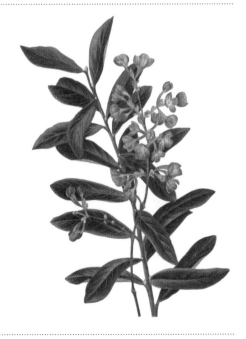

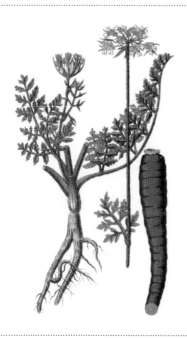

Daucus carota
Carrot

Biennial from Iran with umbrella-like clusters of white flowers in late summer. The wild carrot's wiry roots are red-purple due to the presence of anthocyanins – these have been bred out of the cultivated orange carrot. Prefers rich, well-drained soils in sun.

Part(s) used Root.
Traditional uses Root was eaten to stimulate pituitary gland secretion and to treat threadworms, gout, rheumatism, cystitis and urinary problems. Diuretic properties were considered helpful for kidney complaints.
Medicinal discoveries Root extracts have antibacterial activity which could explain its use for urinary infections.

Descurainia sophia
Flixweed, the wisdom of surgeons

Annual or biennial, naturalized as a weed on waste ground and roadsides in many parts of the world. Occurs in light soils in E. England. Yellow flowers appear in early summer.

Part(s) used Flower, leaf, seed.
Traditional uses Called 'the wisdom of surgeons' because of its healing properties. Flowers and leaves were used to treat chronic coughs, sore throats, asthma, heart problems, fever, dysentery and burns. Seeds were used to make a tonic for fevers, bronchitis, asthma, burns and sciatica. Still used in herbal remedies for toothache and coughs.
Medicinal discoveries Seed extracts shown to have antibacterial activity.

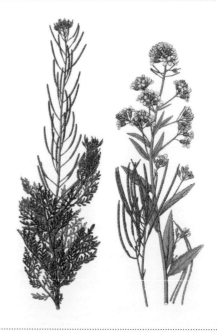

Dipsacus inermis
Perennial teasel

Perennial herb from Asia that grows in woods and near streams. Has prickly stem and leaves, white-yellow to purple flowers in summer to early autumn. Good source of seeds for garden birds. The flower head persists and can be used in floral displays.

Part(s) used Aerial parts.
Traditional uses Used internationally in folk remedies to treat Lyme disease, fibromyalgia, cancer and bone fractures. Used in traditional Chinese medicine as a tonic for liver problems.
Medicinal discoveries Increased interest in studying the plant for leads in the treatment of cancer and Alzheimer's disease.

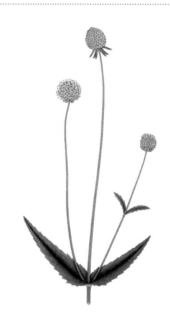

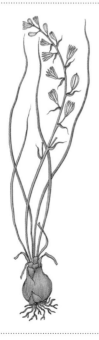

Drimia indica
Indian squill

Spring-flowering, perennial herbaceous grown from bulbs, with long leaves and bell-shaped, white-yellow flowers. Native to Asia and parts of Africa.

Part(s) used Bulb, leaf.
Traditional uses Extracts were used as an expectorant, rubbed on to the soles of the feet to relieve burning sensations, to remove warts and for treating heart problems, bronchitis, asthma, whooping cough and oedema.
Medicinal discoveries Plant contains toxic cardiac glycosides which are strongly diuretic and slow the heartbeat. Scientific studies have supported some of the traditional uses of this plant. It should only be used under professional supervision.

Drynaria roosii
Gu-Sui-Bu

Fern that is distributed in China, Indochina and Thailand.

Part(s) used Rhizome.
Traditional uses Often described by the synonym *Drynaria fortunei*, this traditional Chinese medicine has been used for bone disorders such as osteoporosis as well as for heart problems, inflammatory conditions and rheumatic complaints.
Medicinal discoveries Some studies suggest that rhizome preparations and constituents might promote proliferation of bone cells and bone mineral density. Rhizome constituents might also have oestrogen-like effects. More studies are needed to explore potential benefits for osteoporosis.

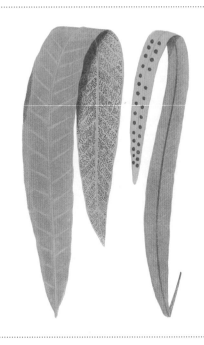

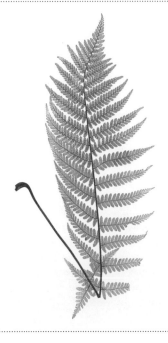

Dryopteris filix-mas
Male fern

Deciduous or semi-evergreen fern that occurs in Eurasia and N. and S. America. Grown in gardens for its attractive foliage, hardiness and drought-resistance. Different cultivars have different leaf and frond shapes.

Part(s) used Rhizome (and frond-base).
Traditional uses Traditionally used as a remedy for tapeworm and liver flukes. Used to relieve pain and inflammation and to lower fever. It was also used to control bleeding and an ointment was applied to wounds.
Medicinal discoveries The male fern is highly toxic so is no longer used for medicinal applications. Some studies suggest it has antifungal properties.

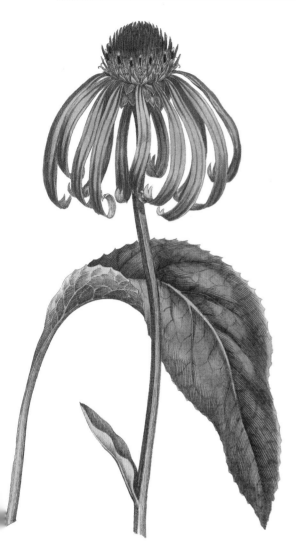

Echinacea purpurea
Echinacea, cone flower

Perennial from the eastern parts of N. America, produces purple daisy-like flowers with a honey fragrance. The flower centres are orange-brown with a prickly appearance, hence the name derived from the Greek *echinose*, meaning hedgehog.

Part(s) used Aerial parts, root.

Traditional uses *Echinacea purpurea*, together with *E. angustifolia* and *E. pallida*, have been used medicinally for centuries for their reputed anti-infective and antitoxin properties. Echinacea preparations were applied as remedies for painful skin conditions, such as boils and wounds, and taken to treat snakebites, mouth inflammations and tonsillitis. They were also thought to alleviate the symptoms of colds, flu and fevers. The root was used for haemorrhoids and diphtheria and was reputed to have aphrodisiac properties.

Medicinal discoveries Current interest in echinacea has focused on its potential to stimulate the immune system, especially to help prevent the onset of colds and flu. Scientific studies revealed that echinacea preparations can modulate the function of the immune system. They also have antiviral, antibacterial, antifungal and anti-inflammatory properties. When echinacea preparations were tested in clinical trials on people, some beneficial effects were reported, suggesting it might help prevent respiratory infections. However, more studies using good-quality echinacea preparations with known chemical constituents are needed to confirm the potential benefits against colds and flu.

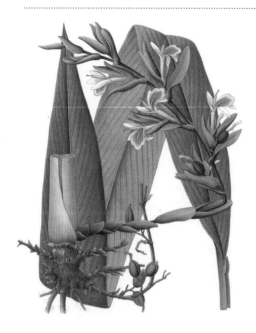

Elettaria cardamomum
Cardamom

Perennial aromatic spice found in S. India and parts of Asia.

Part(s) used Seed.
Traditional uses Seeds when combined with other herbal medicines were used as a 'corrective remedy'. Seeds were considered to produce a 'grateful not fiery warmth' and were a remedy for indigestion, colic and flatulence. They were also reputed to be good for disorders of the head.
Medicinal discoveries Cardamom seeds are used in preparations to relieve flatulence and are also used as a culinary flavouring, adding a warm, spicy-sweetness to food.

Elymus repens
Couch grass

Perennial grass that is native to Europe and Asia. It has creeping rhizomes that will grow in most soils. It is considered an invasive weed but can be used in sandy soils to prevent soil erosion. It flowers in summer.

Part(s) used Leaf, root.
Traditional uses Traditionally used in parts of Europe to treat fever, sore throats, urinary infections, gout and rheumatism. Cats and dogs eat the leaves as an emetic (to cause vomiting). Used by herbalists to treat urinary infections and sore throats.
Medicinal discoveries Rhizomes are valued for their mucilage (gelatinous sap) and experiments have shown that they have anti-inflammatory activity.

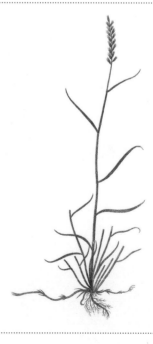

Ephedra distachya
Sea grape, shrubby horsetail

Evergreen shrub with bluish-green stems, occurring from S. Europe to Siberia. Some *Ephedra* species are cultivated as shrubs for ground cover.

Part(s) used Stem.

Traditional uses A traditional Chinese medicine for kidney weakness. *Ephedra* species have been used for coughs, colds and fevers and to alleviate asthma, rashes, hay fever and rheumatic complaints.

Medicinal discoveries *Ephedra* species contain the alkaloids ephedrine and pseudoephedrine, which have been developed as medicines to alleviate nasal congestion, although they can cause adverse effects and their use is restricted.

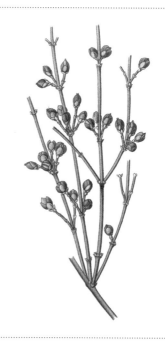

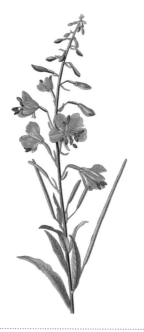

Epilobium angustifolium
Rosebay willowherb

European perennial herb with tall, erect stems bearing willowy leaves topped with pink-purple flowers. Spreads quickly by shallow horizontal roots. Considered a weed as it occurs in waste ground and woodland clearings. Often grown as a bee plant in sheltered or open areas, such as a meadow.

Part(s) used Leaf, root.

Traditional uses Traditionally used to treat whooping cough, asthma, swellings, boils and carbuncles. Poultices were made from the leaves to treat wounds.

Medicinal discoveries Laboratory studies have shown that extracts of the plant have anti-inflammatory activity.

Equisetum arvense
Horsetail

This herbaceous perennial plant from arctic and northern parts of the world was dominant during the Carboniferous age around 300 million years ago. It has fertile spore-bearing stems that are produced in early spring and grow underground. They then whither and the sterile non-reproductive green stems grow and persist through the summer, spreading like a weed to form a dense carpet of foliage.

Part(s) used Aerial parts.

Traditional uses Traditionally used to treat chilblains, conjunctivitis, wounds and skin disorders, to strengthen fingernails, and a gargle for mouth and gum inflammations, for kidney and urinary tract infections, diarrhoea, tuberculosis, flu, haemorrhoids, rheumatism and gout. Still widely used in herbal medicine for the treatment of urinary infections. In traditional Chinese medicine it is used to cool fevers and to treat flu, swellings and haemorrhoids.

Medicinal discoveries Despite the long term use of this plant there is a lack of clinical data to support its uses. However, laboratory studies have shown it has antibacterial activity, and data from research on other species of *Equisetum* has shown that they have diuretic activity. It is not known what factors influence the variation in the chemistry of the plant, which will effect the medicinal properties of the plant.

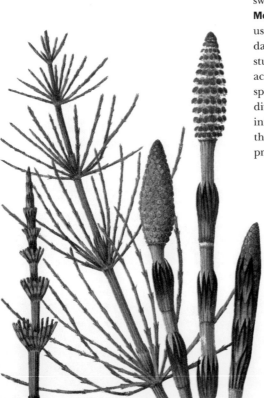

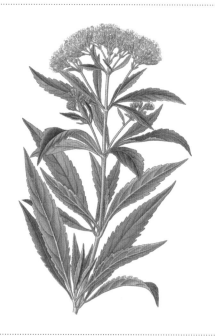

Eupatorium cannabinum
Hemp-agrimony

European herbaceous perennial grown as an ornamental bee plant. Has red stems and mauve-white flowers from summer through to autumn.

Part(s) used Aerial parts, root.
Traditional uses Used as a tonic to clear the blood and to treat flu, fever and jaundice. Externally used to treat minor skin infections, bleeding, bruising and wounds. The root of the plant was used as a laxative and diuretic and to treat constipation. Still used as a homoeopathic tincture for flu.
Medicinal discoveries Plant contains toxic pyrrolizidine alkaloids which have anti-inflammatory and antioxidant properties.

Fagopyrum esculentum
Buckwheat

Annual that produces clusters of fragrant, pink-white flowers followed by edible seeds. Used as a green manure by gardeners.

Part(s) used Aerial parts, hulled seed.
Traditional uses An infusion was used as a remedy for 'St Anthony's fire' and other red rashes associated with infected skin. A poultice of the flour with buttermilk was considered to 'restore the flow of milk in nurses'. The aerial parts are included in herbal preparations for circulation problems.
Medicinal discoveries Hulled seeds have been associated with several potential health benefits, including lowering cholesterol. There is interest in its anticancer, antidiabetic and anti-inflammatory properties.

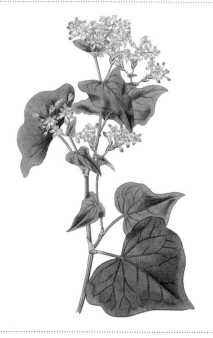

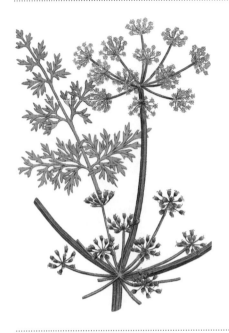

Ferula assa-foetida
Asafoetida

Perennial herb found growing in the deserts of W. Asia, Iran and Afghanistan. It grows in dry, sandy, open sites and produces clusters of green-white summer flowers.

Part(s) used Aerial parts, root.
Traditional uses Used to treat flatulence, constipation, asthma, bronchitis, whooping cough and to aid digestion. In 1918 was used as a remedy in the Spanish influenza pandemic. Used in Ayurvedic medicine to aid digestion and treat blood pressure.
Medicinal discoveries Some scientific data to support its anti-viral uses. A clinical trial supported its use in the treatment of irritable bowel syndrome.

Ficus carica
Fig

Native to the Middle East, found growing on hot, dry soils in scrub and among rocks. Drought tolerant, best grown with the roots contained. Ideal grown against a wall. Will fruit in a warm environment.

Part(s) used Fruit, stem latex.
Traditional uses Fruits traditionally eaten to aid digestion, as a mild laxative, to treat fatigue, haemorrhoids, piles and gout, and applied topically to treat wounds. Latex from stems was used to remove warts and corns. Syrup of figs is still used for the short term relief of occasional constipation.
Medicinal discoveries Laboratory studies have shown that the fig latex and fruits have a wide range of medicinal properties.

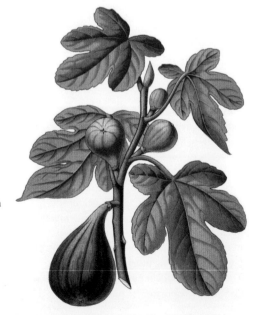

A history of herbals

Written evidence about the medicinal uses of plants goes back 5,000 years to the Sumerians, in southern Mesopotamia, who listed the plants they used on clay tablets. Around 2,500BC in China, oral knowledge about medicinal plants was documented in the herbal *Shennong Bencao Jing* (Shennong's *materia medica* classic). The early use of plants in Indian medicine was documented in classical Sanskrit literature, around 4,000–5,000 years ago.

Within Europe the early herbals were written in Greek or Latin. Pedanius Dioscorides (AD40–90) and Aelius Galenus (AD131–200) were both Greek surgeons employed in the Roman army. Their herbals helped define *materia medica* texts (treatises on medical remedies) and Dioscorides' herbal is considered to be the precursor to all modern pharmacopoeias. Later, Philip van Hohenheim (1491–1541), known as Paracelsus, a Swiss physician and keen gardener, revived some of the concepts developed by Dioscorides and Galenus in the Doctrine of Signatures. He proposed that

'Nature marks each growth…according to its curative benefit'. The appearance of the plant indicated its medicinal use: herbs used to cure jaundice often had yellow flowers, whereas pansies, with their heart-shaped petals, could cure heart problems.

In Britain, monasteries had long been the guardians of herbal medicine: not only did they translate the classical herbals, they also prescribed herbal remedies. In 1597, gardener and herbalist John Gerard published his *The Herball, or generall historie of plantes*, which was a translation of a herbal published in 1554 by the Flemish physician Rembert Dodoen. In 1653, Nicholas Culpeper, a botanist and physician who had an interest in astrology, published *The English Physician* (now known as *Culpeper's Herbal*) in which he reintroduced the links plants and diseases could have to the signs of the zodiac.

In the latter part of the sixteenth century there was an increased understanding of diseases and their treatment. This resulted in a need for more evidence based herbals, resulting in our modern pharmacopoeias.

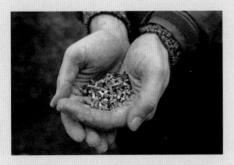

Sliced branches of witch hazel
(*Hamamelis virginiana*)
(see page 98).

Filipendula ulmaria
Meadowsweet, mead-sweet

The common name 'mead-sweet' is thought
to derive from the plant's use in flavouring
mead. It is also known as bridewort, as the
creamy-coloured, cloud-like flowers were
used as wedding decorations. The honey-
almond scent of the flowers intensifies on
drying and it was popular as a strewing herb
to perfume rooms (see page 220).

The scientific name of the genus was once
Spiraea, which is where aspirin, the first
mass-produced drug, gets its name from.
Aspirin was developed from the compound
salicylic acid, which was isolated from
meadowsweet and white willow. Both plants
were used as anti-inflammatories to relieve
the pain of rheumatic joint and muscle
conditions. They were also used for fevers.

Meadowsweet is now used mainly as a herb
for the digestive system, principally as an
antacid for gastric reflux (heartburn)
and to reduce the risk of stomach ulcers
developing. Its anti-inflammatory effects
on the gut may assist in irritable bowel
syndrome (IBS). It is also used to relieve
diarrhoea. There is very little recent
scientific research into the medicinal effects
of meadowsweet.

Grow In moist, fertile soil, preferably clay
or loam, in full sun to partial shade.
Harvest Pick flowering tops on a sunny day
in summer; leave outside so any insects fly
away. Pick leaves in spring before flowering.
Caution Should not be used by people with
salicylate sensitivity.

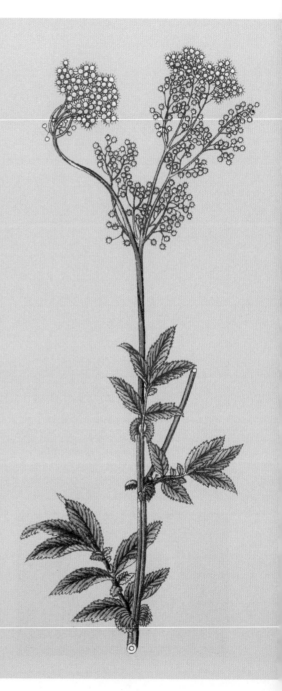

Meadowsweet tincture

Tinctures are an alcoholic extract of a plant that concentrates and preserves its active chemicals. Take 5 ml (1 teaspoon) mixed with water, two to three times a day before meals, to relieve the symptoms of acid reflux and IBS. Use in place of almond essence when baking cakes and puddings.

50 g (1¾ oz) dried meadowsweet flowers

300 ml (10½ fl oz) brandy 25%–40% alcohol

You will also need: bowl; measuring jug; sterilized, lidded jar; wide-necked funnel or cone made of paper; clean muslin; sterilized bottle with stopper

1. Break flowers up into small pieces in a bowl then transfer to the sterilized jar using a wide-necked funnel or cone of paper.

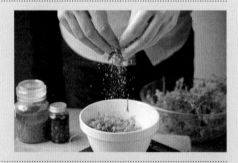

2. Add the brandy to the jar, screw on the lid and shake to combine. Top up with brandy to cover the flowers.

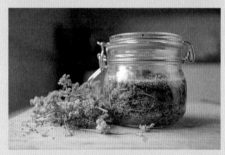

3. Leave to infuse for one month in a cool, dark place. Turn the jar every two to three days, topping up with brandy to keep the flowers covered. After a month, strain through a muslin-lined funnel into a sterilized bottle and seal. Will keep for two years.

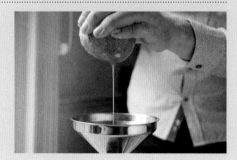

Foeniculum vulgare
Fennel

The twelfth-century Benedictine abbess Hildegard von Bingen described fennel as 'beneficial for anybody, whether healthy or ill. . . it makes a person happy and brings to him a gentle heat and good perspiration, and makes his digestion good'. She also recommended it mixed with other herbs for ulcers, clouded vision, poor sleep and as a wash for sore eyes. Fennel seeds are commonly eaten after a meal in India to freshen the breath and aid digestion. They are also recommended in European herbals to reduce flatulence and to lose weight.

Fennel 'seeds' are actually fruits that contain two seeds. They are reported to work as an aphrodisiac and enlarge breasts, and are still widely used to stimulate milk production by nursing mothers in both Europe and China. They contain phytoestrogens, chemicals similar to the sex hormone oestrogen, which may contribute to these traditional uses.

Fennel seeds are used in the production of many spirits, including absinthe and ouzo, contributing to the clouding effect when water is added to these drinks. References do not agree on whether fennel stimulates or suppresses the appetite, and drinks made from it are used as both *aperitifs* and *digestifs*.

Grow Plant in full sun in well-drained soil. Probably originating in the Mediterranean, it is widely cultivated and considered invasive in California, New Zealand and Australia.
Harvest Wait until the seeds turn brown before harvesting.

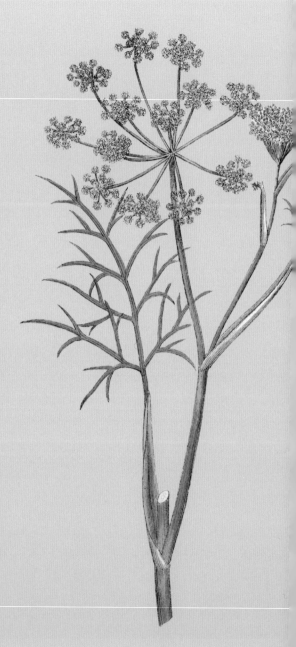

Fennel tincture

You can decide for yourself the effect of fennel on the appetite by making this simple infused spirit at home. Take 5 ml (1 teaspoon) mixed with water twice a day to improve digestion and reduce flatulence.

40 g (1½ oz) fennel seeds

200 ml (7 fl oz) vodka or other non-flavoured 40% spirit

You will also need: scales; pestle and mortar; a sterilized, lidded jar; wide-necked funnel or cone of paper; measuring jug; muslin; small dropper bottles

1. Grind fennel seeds with a pestle and mortar or spice grinder, then pour into the jar using a wide-necked funnel or cone of paper. Pour over the vodka and close lid.

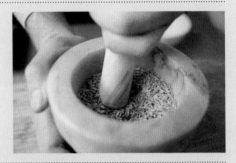

2. Leave to infuse for one month, turning every two to three days.

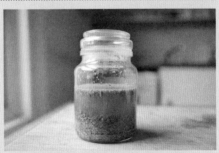

3. Strain through a muslin-lined funnel into individual dropper bottles. Will keep for up to two years.

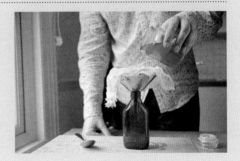

Forsythia suspensa
Weeping forsythia

Elegant, hardy, deciduous shrub from China with spreading, pendulous branches and abundant golden-yellow spring flowers.

Part(s) used Fruit, leaf, root.
Traditional uses One of the fifty fundamental herbs used in traditional Chinese medicine. Fruit used for intestinal worms, boils and skin infections and to control menstruation. Leaves were used for sore throats, high blood pressure, breast cancer and diarrhoea. Roots were used for colds, fever and jaundice.
Medicinal discoveries Its anti-inflammatory, antitumour and antibacterial properties have been confirmed. Clinical trials are needed to evaluate the traditional uses.

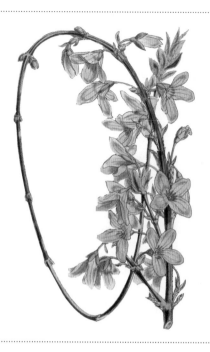

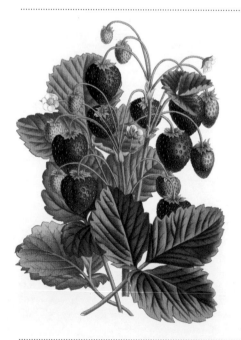

Fragaria vesca
Wild strawberry

Perennial found in grasslands and woods in Europe and N. America. Produces white flowers in spring followed by small, red, edible fruits. Good ground cover plant.

Part(s) used Fruit, leaf.
Traditional uses Used in folk medicine as a laxative and diuretic. Berries were reputed to cure gout and leaves were considered good for dysentery. Culpeper (see page 81) claimed the plant as being 'singularly good for the healing of many ills'.
Medicinal discoveries The fruit has antioxidant properties and has been suggested to have anticancer and anti-blood clotting effects. Leaf preparations have been shown to mediate effects on the heart.

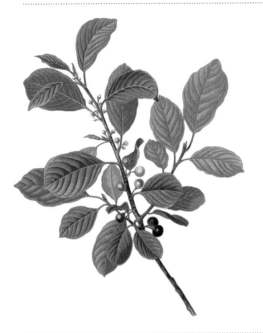

Frangula alnus
Alder buckthorn

A native of Europe and parts of Asia, this tree grows in wet boggy soils, in hedgerows and heathland and by rivers. Brown bark turns yellow when exposed to air. Small, star-shaped, green-white flowers in early summer followed by red to black berries.

Part(s) used Bark (inner).
Traditional uses Used for skin irritations, as a purgative and to treat diabetes.
Medicinal discoveries Contains compounds called anthraquinone glycosides that are associated with its use as a laxative. Clinical data support its use for the short-term treatment of constipation and for intestinal evacuation before X-rays.

Fumaria officinalis
Fumitory

Herbaceous annual plant native to Europe with grey-green leaves and small, pink, purple-tipped flowers on stalks throughout spring and summer.

Part(s) used Leaf, latex-like sap.
Traditional uses Used to treat skin and eye conditions, cleanse the kidneys, soothe headaches and muscle and gall-bladder pain. Used by herbalists for a range of conditions including indigestion, gall bladder and liver problems.
Medicinal discoveries Latex-like sap is rich in isoquinoline alkaloids which can be toxic. Latex should be treated with great care. Laboratory studies support some of the traditional uses but clinical data are lacking.

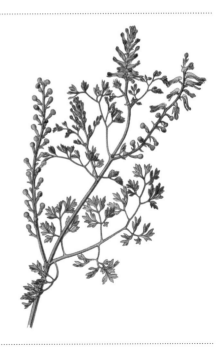

Galium aparine
Cleavers, goosegrass

Native to Europe, N. Africa and Asia, now naturalized in most parts of the world as a weed. Common in hedgerows, field margins and waste areas in a garden. The creeping stems, which are covered with hooked hairs, branch and grow along the ground and over other plants. It has tiny, star-shaped, white-green flowers from early spring to summer.

Part(s) used Aerial parts.

Traditional uses Long history of traditional use as a poultice to treat skin ailments including wounds, burns, eczema and psoriasis. Extracts were used as a diuretic, to help reduce fever, and as a tonic for insomnia, glandular fever, tonsillitis, cystitis and cancer. As a pulp, it has been used to relieve poisonous bites and stings. Herbalists prescribed it for a range of conditions including as a poultice to treat leg wounds not responding to other treatments, especially in immune-suppressed patients. To make a poultice, fresh material is used and applied to the affected area.

Medicinal discoveries Plant shown to contain a range of compounds called coumarins, iridoids and flavonoids that could explain some of the medicinal uses. Further laboratory and clinical data is needed to fully evaluate the profile of compounds needed in an effective extract.

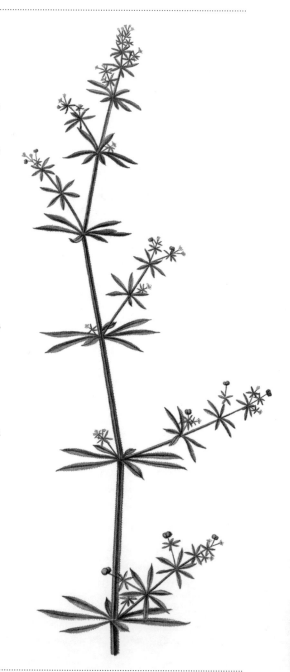

Gardenia jasminoides
Gardenia

Evergreen tree or shrub from China and Japan with glossy leaves and large, fragrant, white flowers in summer and autumn.

Part(s) used Fruit.
Traditional uses In Asia, gardenia was used to decrease swellings in rheumatoid arthritis as well as to treat anxiety, agitation, depression and insomnia and to detoxify the blood, stop bleeding and promote healing. In the West, it has also been used to reduce inflammation. Some aromatherapists prescribe gardenia oil for anxiety and nervous tension due to its calming effect.
Medicinal discoveries Recent research has shown the plant may have antidepressant effects.

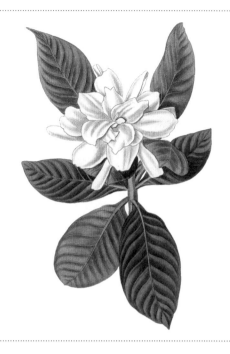

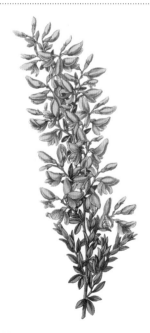

Genista tinctoria
Dyer's greenweed

Deciduous shrub with numerous cultivars bred as a garden ornamental. Yellow pea-like flowers in spring to early summer are followed by long, shiny green seed pods. Grows in poor, well-drained soil in full sun. Useful plant that will fix nitrogen in the soil.

Part(s) used Aerial parts of plant in flower.
Traditional uses As a diuretic, emetic and to treat circulatory problems, dropsy, rheumatism and gout. Still used for various complaints, including skin diseases.
Medicinal discoveries The isoflavone compound called genistein was isolated from this plant in 1899; scientifically it has been shown to have a wide range of pharmacological properties.

Gentiana lutea
Gentian, yellow gentian

Herbaceous perennial with star-shaped, yellow flowers that occurs widely in temperate regions.

Part(s) used Root.

Traditional uses The root was prepared as a bitter tonic considered useful in states of exhaustion and debility. It was reputed to aid the digestion and help the appetite. It was considered a remedy for 'female weakness', hysteria and to combat fevers. The seventeenth-century herbalist Nicholas Culpeper (see page 81) claimed gentian 'comforts the heart and preserves it against faintings and swoonings'. He also considered that native gentians in Britain 'have been proved by the experience of divers physicians not to be a whit inferior in virtue to that which comes from beyond the sea'. The root was a remedy to counteract worms and for 'the bitings of mad dogs and venomous beasts'.

Medicinal discoveries There has been much interest in the use of gentian to relieve digestive complaints and some studies suggest it might help symptoms of indigestion and heartburn (dyspepsia). Furthermore, it might be of some use for loss of appetite and constipation. It has also been studied for its potential to treat inflamed gastrointestinal problems and for its antioxidant, anti-inflammatory and anticancer effects.

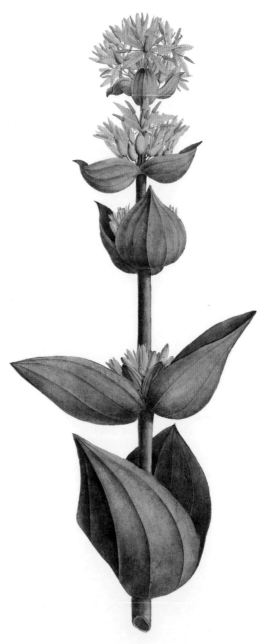

Ginkgo biloba
Ginkgo, maidenhair tree

A native of China that has been cultivated in Europe for over 300 years. Dating back 270 million years, ginkgo is the oldest living tree species and is often referred to as a living fossil. Its leaves are unique among seed plants as they are fan-shaped with veins radiating out into the leaf blade; they turn saffron yellow in autumn. Good resistance to wind and snow damage but doesn't like shade.

Part(s) used Leaf, seed.
Traditional uses Use of seeds in traditional Chinese medicine can be traced to 2800BC for treating coughs, asthma and bladder disorders. Leaves were used to treat cardiovascular problems, muscular degeneration and altitude sickness.

Medicinal discoveries Leaf extracts that contain 22–27 per cent of the active compounds called flavonoid glycosides have been marketed in parts of Europe since the 1960s as a dietary supplement to enhance cognitive function. Clinical studies on the use of these extracts for the treatment of dementia and Alzheimer's disease have shown mixed results. These differences could be due to variations in the levels in the extracts of the active compounds. Currently, there is increased interest in the contribution these compounds could play in the use of ginkgo extracts for treating cardiovascular conditions.

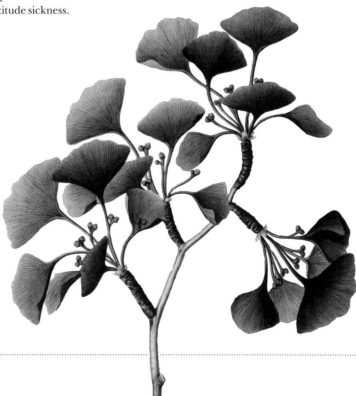

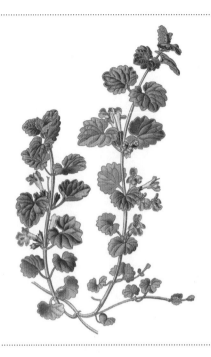

Glechoma hederacea
Ground ivy

Aromatic, evergreen, creeping perennial from Europe and S.W. Asia. In spring the plant produces blue-violet, funnel-shaped flowers. It prefers moist shade but will tolerate sun. Often found growing in lawns, it will survive frequent mowing.

Part(s) used Aerial parts.
Traditional uses Used in Europe to treat eye problems, tinnitus, kidney, liver, respiratory and urinary disease and as a tonic for fever, colds and coughs. Herbalists prescribe it as a mild expectorant and digestive.
Medicinal discoveries Laboratory studies support its traditional uses but there is a lack of clinical data.

Glycine max
Soya bean; soy bean

Annual originating from Asia that produces white, lilac or pink clusters of flowers.

Part(s) used Seed.
Traditional uses Mainly used for food. Records of soy cultivation date back to the eleventh century BC in China.
Medicinal discoveries Seeds contain compounds called isoflavones that have oestrogen-like properties. There has been much interest in the use of soy isoflavones to alleviate menopausal symptoms and to maintain heart health. Soy isoflavones have also been of interest for cancer prevention and to aid memory. Soy milk is used as an alternative for cow's milk.

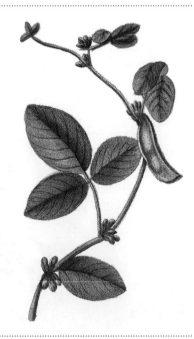

Traditional systems of medicine

The healing or poisonous properties of plants have been extensively explored by humans for centuries. This traditional knowledge has been passed on for many generations and recorded in ancient texts, *materia medicas* (treatise on medical remedies) and pharmacopoeias (provide standards for the identity and quality of medicines). These records give us clues about the medicinal uses of plants, and often include plant descriptions and analytical tests to identify them.

Records of traditional Chinese medicine (TCM) date back almost 5,000 years. These ancient scripts include the compendium *Shennong Bencao Jing*, which was compiled over 2,000 years ago and documents over 300 medicinal preparations. The current Pharmacopoeia of the People's Republic of China describes over 2,000 TCM remedies. The principles of this medical system are based on restoring the balance of the body, the *yin* and the *yang*, and adjusting the body's energy flow, the *qi*. TCM uses herbs, other medicinal substances, acupuncture and dietary factors. The herbs used are often combined and prepared as decoctions.

One of the most famous is ginseng (*Panax ginseng*) root, which has been used for over 2,000 years for many conditions, including those associated with old age. TCM is now becoming popular world wide, including in the UK and North America.

Other traditional practices of medicine from Asia, particularly India, include Ayurvedic, Siddha, and Unani. Ayurvedic medicine is an ancient system of healthcare that has been practised for over 5,000 years. It involves herbal medicines, minerals, diet and meditation. One of the earliest written texts, the *Charaka Samhita*, dates back to 300BC and is considered central to the modern-day practice of Ayurvedic medicine. Widely used Ayurvedic herbs are the *Rasayanas*, which are thought to increase longevity, and include Indian ginseng (*Withania somnifera*). Ayurvedic medicine is increasing in popularity as a holistic approach to health.

Numerous other traditional systems of medicine have been practised throughout the world, and for many populations, plants remain an important source of medicines.

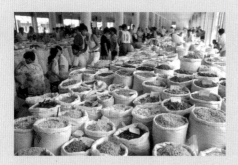

A vast range of traditional
Chinese herbal medicines may be
found in local markets in China.

Glycyrrhiza glabra
Liquorice

The name *Glycyrrhiza* derives from the ancient Greek 'glykys' (sweet) and 'rhiza' (root). The root, which can be up to 50 times sweeter than sugar, is an important herb in many medical traditions. It is often used in remedies to mask the bitter flavour of other herbs. Liquorice was traditionally understood as having a demulcent action, helping to soothe inflammation and irritation by forming a protective coating – hence its use for sore throats and for acid reflux. It is also prescribed by herbalists as an expectorant, helping to expel mucus from the lungs. In laboratory tests, extracts were active against several viruses, and also showed promise in the treatment of mouth ulcers. Liquorice is also being investigated for its effect on protecting the liver. In Japan it has been used to treat chronic hepatitis C.

A Dutch doctor in the 1940s noticed his patients making a swift recovery from stomach ulcers after taking a liquorice preparation from a local pharmacy. He discovered the chemical glycyrrhizin, which was developed into carbenoxolone – the main drug prescribed for stomach and duodenal ulcers in the 1960s.

Grow Needs a sheltered site in light or full sun in an alkaline, sandy but moist soil. Light blue-violet flowers appear in summer.
Harvest Pick rhizomes off the main tap root in early autumn, alternating sides each year. Use fresh or wash, then dry and store.
Caution Liquorice must not be taken for longer than four weeks without medical supervision. Must not be used by anyone with hypertension or other heart problems. Always talk to a pharmacist before taking.

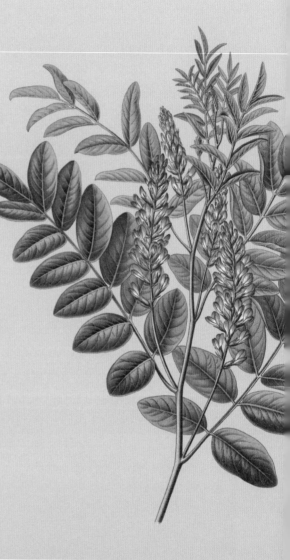

Liquorice sweets

A traditional way to take herbal medicine for a sore throat is to combine the ingredients with sugar to make sweets. Suck up to three sweets a day to relieve a hoarse, dry or infected throat, for up to five days running. The mixture tends to bubble when heated, so use a deep saucepan and keep an eye on it at all times.

1 kg (2 lb 3 oz) icing sugar

50 g (1¾ oz) dried liquorice roots

10 g (½ oz) aniseeds

250 ml (9 fl oz) water

500 g (18 oz) caster sugar

You will also need: baking tray; small bottle; deep sauce pan; heatproof measuring jug; sugar thermometer; pastry brush; airtight tin

1. Begin by making moulds for the sweets. Spoon the icing sugar into a baking tray and flatten with your hands to form a layer about 3 cm (1¼ in) deep. Using the base of the bottle, make sweet-sized indentations in the sugar.

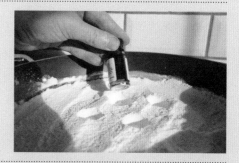

2. Put the roots, seeds and water in a deep saucepan, cover with a lid and simmer for 15 minutes. Turn off the heat and leave for one hour. When cool, strain the liquid into a measuring jug. Dissolve the liquid and sugar together over a medium heat; for each 100 ml (3½ fl oz) of liquid add 200 g (7 oz) caster sugar. Wipe away any sugar from the sides of the pan using a wet pastry brush.

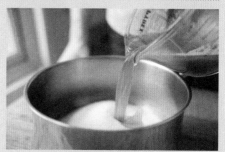

3. Place a sugar thermometer in the pan. Bring to the boil and watch closely as it bubbles up until it reaches 150°C/300°F; 'hard crack' temperature. Transfer the mixture into a measuring jug, then quickly pour into the icing sugar moulds. Leave to harden. Store in an airtight tin for up to one year.

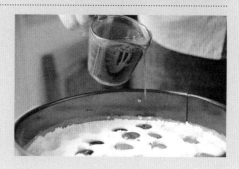

Gossypium hirsutum
Cotton

Native to Central and S. America, this shrubby plant has large, white, cup-shaped flowers. The seed-bearing capsules, called 'bolls', are covered in soft hairs which are spun to produce cotton. Needs sun to flower.

Part(s) used Fruit, root.
Traditional uses Roots were used as a 'female medication' to ease birth and regulate menstruation. Also taken for diarrhoea, dysentery and asthma. Roots were chewed to relieve stomach ache. Fruit was used to treat fibroids and cancer.
Medicinal discoveries The compound gossypol, which is isolated from the cotton plant, reduces sperm count. In Asia it is prescribed as a male contraceptive.

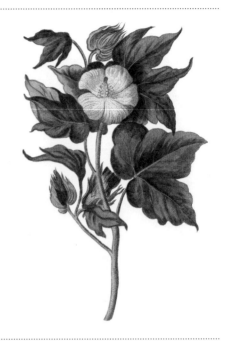

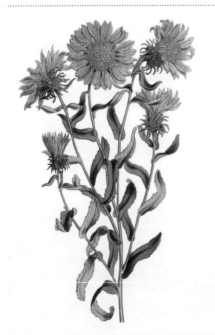

Grindelia hirsutula
Grindelia, gum plant

Annual, or sometimes perennial, from drier regions of N. and S. America, which produces resinous leaves. *G. squarrosa* is from western and central regions of North America.

Part(s) used Flowering aerial parts.
Traditional uses *G. hirsutula* and *G. squarrosa* were traditional remedies for respiratory complaints, such as asthma and bronchitis, and inflamed skin conditions.
Medicinal discoveries Preparations have shown anti-inflammatory properties and have been explored for their potential to alleviate allergic skin reactions caused by contact with poison ivy (*Toxicodendron* species). Components of the resin have a repellent effect on aphids.

Herbalists today

Herbal medicine is a living tradition that continues to attract interest. A significant number of people still train and practise as herbalists across Europe and North America. However, they face a variety of challenges in practising due to the particular legal situations in their countries. The two main challenges are: whether the law allows them to carry out medical consultations, and whether they can dispense herbal medicines.

Recently in the European Union (EU) legislation was enacted to regulate the safety of herbal medicines. Each herbal product must first be licensed to enable it to be sold over the counter to the general public. This has meant that only plants that have been shown to have a tradition of use within the EU can be licensed. Manufacturers must also meet quality control regulations in their supply and manufacture. This results in a situation in some countries, such as Portugal, where it is possible to consult, but not dispense directly. Herbalists have to recommend products available over the counter, which can limit the range of herbs they can choose from.

In other countries dispensing is possible, but only within certain limits and if certain criteria are met. In Britain and Ireland, the government has recommended self-regulation, meaning it is legal to offer a consultation as a herbalist and dispense herbal medicines, though some medicines are restricted. In Germany a qualification must be passed to practice in a range of alternative therapies, including herbal medicine.

In the USA, regulation differs state by state, but generally only conventionally trained doctors are allowed to diagnose and treat diseases. Herbalists use their constitutional right to free speech to give people information about their health, whilst adhering to the legal restrictions on dispensing. The quality control of herbal medicines is also strictly regulated. There are campaigns to give herbalists more freedom at the state level.

Despite the challenges they face, herbalists in Europe and the USA are using creative ways to continue to give advice about the use of herbal medicines and provide access to prepared herbal medicines whilst staying in line with the law.

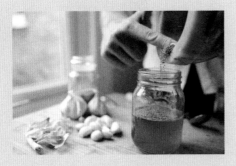

Preparing a garlic oxymel (see recipe page 21). Regulations on preparing and dispensing herbal remedies vary between countries.

Hamamelis virginiana
Witch hazel

Found growing in N.E. America, witch hazel was used by Native North Americans, most commonly as a decoction of the bark or a poultice of the leaves to treat skin sores and inflammation, muscle aches, diarrhoea and coughs. European colonists learned these uses from the indigenous population.

Witch hazel has an antioxidant action and, as with many tree barks, it is high in chemicals called tannins. These chemicals, which act to constrict proteins, are named after their use in tanning leather. This sensation of tightening and drying, known as astringency, can be experienced in red wines that are high in tannins. This effect is useful in small amounts for bleeding and extracts of the bark are applied for haemorrhoids, as an after shave, and for small cuts. The astringency explains why the bark was used internally to treat diarrhoea and dysentery. Witch hazel is also used for bruises and varicose veins. A water distilled from the bark is widely used as a make-up remover and skin toner.

Small studies have found some evidence that lotions made from witch hazel can reduce skin inflammation from nappy rash and sunburn. Several studies show witch hazel ointments can significantly reduce the symptoms of haemorrhoids. A tea made from both the leaf and bark can be an effective mouth gargle for inflamed gums.

Grow Needs a free-draining soil in sun (shade makes plants straggly). Protect young plants from hard frosts. Water during dry spells.
Harvest Pick leaves while they are green. Cut twigs in autumn, ideally when in flower.

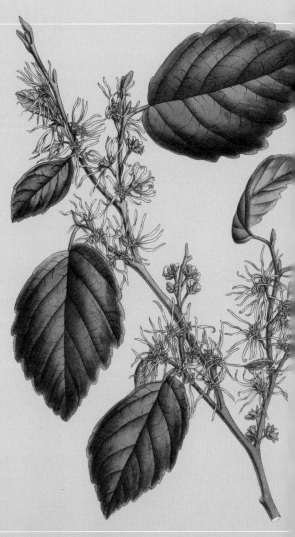

Witch hazel water

Traditionally used as a skin toner, aftershave or for grazes; spray directly on to skin when required. The addition of vodka helps preserve the water-based decoction.

50 g (1¾ oz) witch hazel twigs

300 ml (10 fl oz) water

Around 50 ml (1¾fl oz) vodka

You will also need: bowl; secateurs; large pan; clean muslin; funnel; sterilized bottles or spray bottles

1. Remove the flowers from the twigs and set aside. Using secateurs, slice the twigs into small pieces into a large pan. Pour over the water.

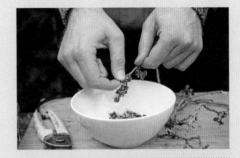

2. Bring to the boil, cover the pan and simmer for one hour. Remove from the heat, add the flowers and vodka and leave overnight to steep.

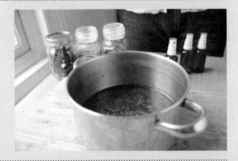

3. Filter through a muslin-lined funnel into sterilized bottles or spray bottles. The infused water will keep for up to six months.

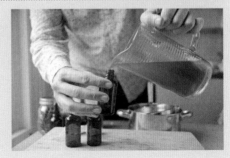

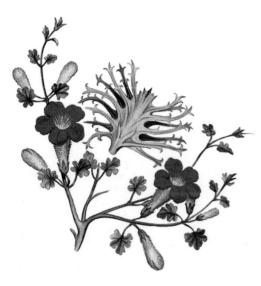

Harpagophytum procumbens
Devil's claw

Trailing perennial from southern Africa that produces crimson or purple trumpet-shaped flowers with thorny fruits.

Part(s) used Secondary root tuber.
Traditional uses Prepared as a tonic to aid digestion and to relieve rheumatic conditions and muscle pains. It was considered to have diuretic and sedative properties.
Medicinal discoveries Modern interest has focused on the anti-inflammatory and pain-relieving properties of extracts. Preparations have been investigated for their potential to alleviate symptoms in arthritic conditions and back pain. Although some studies suggest it has some benefits, more research is needed.

Hedeoma pulegioides
American pennyroyal, squaw mint

Annual that occurs in woods in N.E. America. Its leaves have a mint-like aroma.

Part(s) used Whole plant.
Traditional uses Used by Native North Americans for fevers, headaches, colds and menstrual cramps. It was thought to stimulate the uterus and thus induce abortion. It was also used to aid digestion and was reputed to act as an expectorant.
Medicinal discoveries There are few scientific studies on pennyroyal. Plants and the essential oil, in particular, have been associated with toxic effects. The oil has been used as an insect repellent and in some cleaning products.

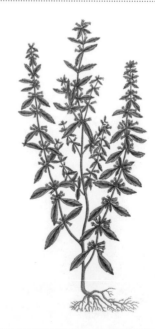

Hedera helix
Ivy

Popular evergreen, leafy, climber that thrives in shady places. Ideal groundcover plant or for growing over walls and outbuildings. Many cultivars are available, including variegated forms.

Part(s) used Leaf.
Traditional uses As an anti-inflammatory and antimicrobial. Also taken for respiratory disorders and as an expectorant for coughs.
Medicinal discoveries Laboratory studies have shown that the saponin compounds in the leaves have antibacterial activity. Nano-particles from the aerial rootlets have also been studied for their use in sunscreens.

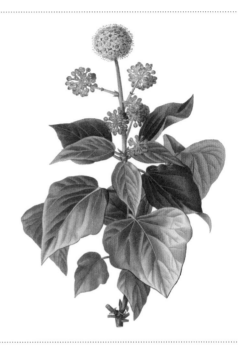

Helianthus annuus
Sunflower

An annual native to the Americas, the sunflower does best in full sun and fertile, moist but well-drained soil. Easy to grow from seed. The stem height, colour and number of flower heads varies among cultivars.

Part(s) used Flower head with seed, leaf.
Traditional uses Leaves were used as a diuretic, as an expectorant and to treat fevers. Leaf poultice was used to treat sores and insect bites. Flower heads with seed used to treat malaria, stomach and pulmonary problems, coughs, colds and rheumatism.
Medicinal discoveries Leaves contain compounds, such as quercetin, that have anti-inflammatory and antiviral properties.

Helleborus niger
Christmas rose, black hellebore

Evergreen perennial from regions in
Germany and Italy. Produces white or
pink flowers in midwinter.

Part(s) used Rhizome.
Traditional uses The rhizome was reputed
to induce abortions and stimulate the
immune system. Preparations were used for
heart problems despite being considered
dangerous. Some homeopathic preparations
use hellebores.
Medicinal discoveries Preparations of
hellebore rhizomes have been investigated
for potential effects on the immune system,
although more studies are needed to
confirm these actions. Harmful if ingested,
can cause skin irritation.

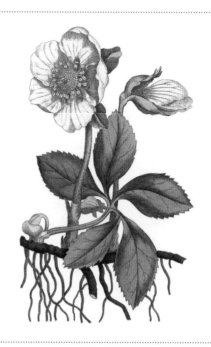

Hepatica nobilis
American liverwort, kidneywort

Small, semi-evergreen perennial with
blue-purple or white-pink flowers. Found in
European woodlands; however, extensive
shade hinders the plant's flowering.

Part(s) used Whole plant.
Traditional uses In the ancient Doctrine
of Signatures, it was a remedy for liver
disorders. The herbalist Culpeper (see page
81) claimed 'it fortifies the liver... and makes
it impregnable'. It was used for digestive
complaints and to promote healing. Other
historical uses were for coughs and lung
problems, including consumption.
Medicinal discoveries Scientific studies that
explore the potential modern uses of the
American liverwort are lacking.

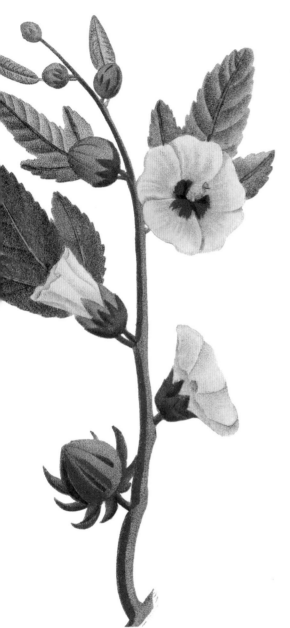

Hibiscus sabdariffa
Hibiscus, East India sorrel plant

Short-lived perennial (often annual) shrubby plant native to W. Africa. Produces white to pale yellow flowers with a dark red calyx. Frost tender, will grow in most soils but must be well drained and in a sheltered spot in direct sun. Potted plants should be watered and fed regularly.

Part(s) used Calyx, leaf, root, seed.
Traditional uses Calyxes used in folk medicine as a diuretic, mild laxative, to relieve coughs, as a remedy for biliousness and for the treatment of hypertension and inflammatory conditions. Leaves were used to treat cracks in the feet, boils, ulcers and wounds. Seeds were reported to have diuretic properties and roots were used to treat stomach problems.
Medicinal discoveries Laboratory studies have shown that the calyxes have high levels of antioxidant activity and there is increased interest in the antimicrobial activity of hibiscus extracts as well as the use of extracts and compounds derived from hibiscus in treating atherosclerosis, liver disease, cancer, diabetes and other metabolic disorders. Health drinks containing hibiscus extracts have become increasingly popular, although any health claims should be treated with caution.

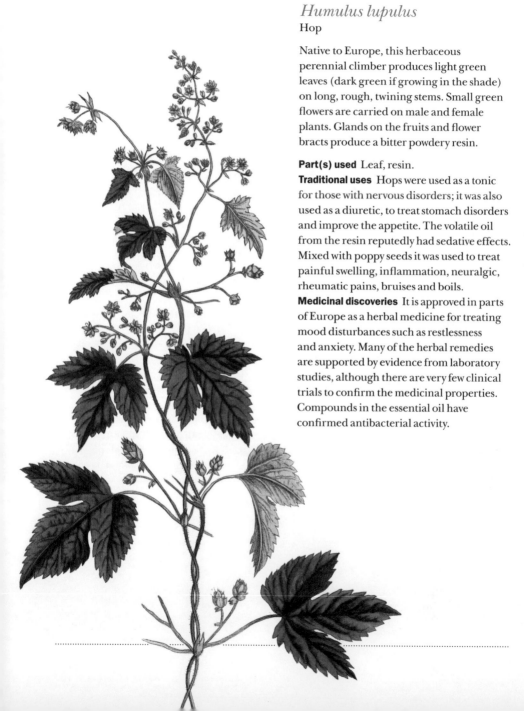

Humulus lupulus
Hop

Native to Europe, this herbaceous perennial climber produces light green leaves (dark green if growing in the shade) on long, rough, twining stems. Small green flowers are carried on male and female plants. Glands on the fruits and flower bracts produce a bitter powdery resin.

Part(s) used Leaf, resin.

Traditional uses Hops were used as a tonic for those with nervous disorders; it was also used as a diuretic, to treat stomach disorders and improve the appetite. The volatile oil from the resin reputedly had sedative effects. Mixed with poppy seeds it was used to treat painful swelling, inflammation, neuralgic, rheumatic pains, bruises and boils.

Medicinal discoveries It is approved in parts of Europe as a herbal medicine for treating mood disturbances such as restlessness and anxiety. Many of the herbal remedies are supported by evidence from laboratory studies, although there are very few clinical trials to confirm the medicinal properties. Compounds in the essential oil have confirmed antibacterial activity.

Hydrangea arborescens
Wild hydrangea, seven bark

Deciduous shrub from E. America that produces clusters of cream-white flowers in late summer fading to green.

Part(s) used Leaf, root.
Traditional uses The root has a long history of use for urinary disorders and decoctions were a remedy to relieve kidney stones and bladder irritations. The root was also used for rheumatic complaints. The leaves were considered to be purgative and diuretic.
Medicinal discoveries The root has been of some interest for alleviating urinary stones and other urinary disorders, although more studies are needed for verification. There has been concern about possible side-effects associated with the herbal use of hydrangea.

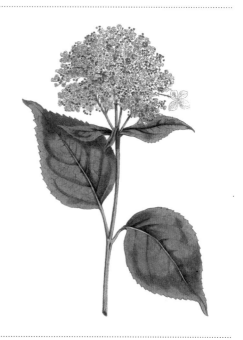

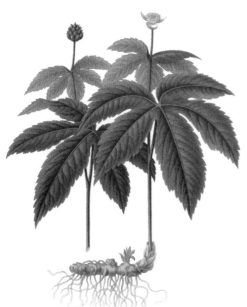

Hydrastis canadensis
Goldenseal

Perennial native to Canada and America, grows in full or partial shade, prefers moist soil. Has a characteristic yellow knotted rhizome and inconspicuous flowers in late spring. Fruits are single and raspberry like.

Part(s) used Root.
Traditional uses Used by the Cherokee Native N. Americans for a wide range of ailments including cancer. In the West it was considered a heal-all and used as an antiseptic, diuretic, laxative and tonic, and for disorders affecting the ears, eyes, nose, intestines, stomach, throat and vagina.
Medicinal discoveries Roots contain isoquinoline alkaloids; these compounds could explain many of the traditional uses.

Hypericum perforatum
St John's wort

This bright perennial begins to flower in June around the feast of St John (24 June). Traditionally this day was marked by lighting fires into which St John's wort was thrown to protect against evil spirits. In France it was known as *chasse-diable*, 'devil chaser'.

The herb can make some people sensitive to sunlight when it is taken internally. When used topically as an oil or cream it has an anti-inflammatory and antioxidant effect; it helps relieve sunburn, mild burns and bruises; it is also a treatment for nerve pain.

St John's wort is one of the most studied herbal medicines in the past twenty years, with the focus being on its antidepressant action. Clinical trials have shown it can be beneficial in treating mild to moderate depression and it is licensed for this purpose in the EU. There is also evidence to support its use for anxiety and seasonal affective disorder (S.A.D.). Recent studies indicate action in stimulating immune cells, promoting repair and antibacterial effects – all three are needed for wound healing. Research has also shown it can increase the rate that the liver processes certain medications (see caution, below).

Grow Will grow in full sun to partial shade in moist but well-drained soil.
Harvest In summer, gather the whole plant while it is in flower.
Caution Check with a pharmacist or health professional before taking internally with other medications, and do not take alongside contraceptive pills.

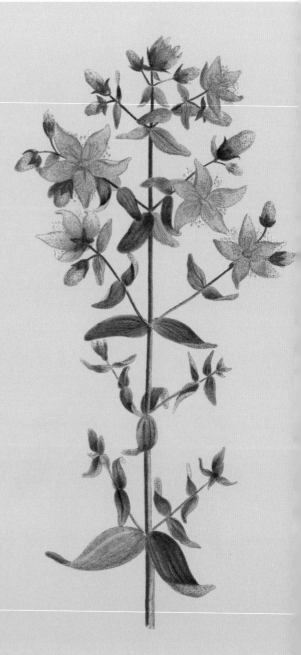

St John's wort sun-infused oil

Many herbs can be infused in oil to make a remedy; the oil can be mixed into creams and balms. St John's wort oil is traditionally used for relieving the symptoms of nerve pain and sunburn. Apply to affected area two to three times a day.

50 g (1¾ oz) fresh flowering tops of St John's wort, left in the sun for a day to dry slightly

300 ml (10 fl oz) almond oil

Vitamin E oil

You will also need: scales; blender; measuring jug; sterilized, lidded wide-necked jar; clean muslin; funnel; sterilized bottle with stopper

1. Press the flowering tops into the jar and pour over the almond oil.

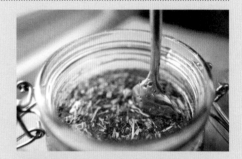

2. Place the jar on a sunny windowsill, every two or three days giving the mixture a gentle shake. Add more almond oil if the level needs topping up – the plant material should stay covered.

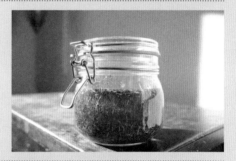

3. After four weeks the oil should have taken on the hue of caramel or a light amber red. Strain through a muslin-lined funnel into a sterilized bottle. Store in a cool place away from light and use within three months. To extend shelf life, add three drops of vitamin E oil and store in the fridge.

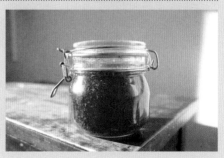

Hyssopus officinalis
Hyssop

Versatile aromatic herb from S. Europe
and the Middle East with dark green, linear
leaves and whorls of blue-white fragrant
flowers in summer. Can be grown as a low
hedge or in borders.

Part(s) used Aerial parts.
Traditional uses Valued as an antiseptic
and for treating respiratory and stomach
problems. Used in preparations for eye
drops and mouthwashes. Still used for
gastrointestinal problems.
Medicinal discoveries Some of the plant's
traditional uses can be explained by the
compounds thujone and phenol that occur
in its essential oil.

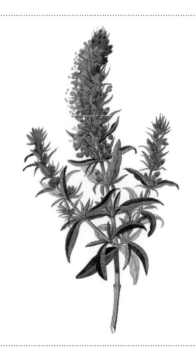

Illicium verum
Star anise

Evergreen shrub or tree from China and
Vietnam. White-yellow flowers turn pink-
red, followed by star-shaped fruits.

Part(s) used Fruit.
Traditional uses Reputed to have warming
and stimulating properties and was taken
to aid digestion and relieve pain. The fruit
was also used as an expectorant remedy for
coughs and catarrhs. The fruit is still a widely
used culinary spice and the essential oil from
the fruit is used in aromatherapy.
Medicinal discoveries Star anise is a source
of a chemical called shikimic acid, which
is used in the manufacture of the anti-
influenza drug oseltamivir.

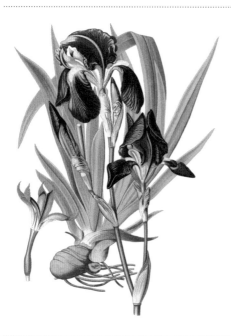

Iris x germanica
Flag iris, orris, German iris

Mediterranean perennial with white and purple flowers. *Iris versicolor* (blue flag) is native to N. America and has purple and yellow-veined flowers.

Part(s) used Rhizome.
Traditional uses Rhizome juice was reputed to treat dropsy when it was combined with wine. Made into a traditional remedy, rhizomes were given for coughs and catarrhs and were applied to wounds. *I. versicolor* (blue flag) was used by Native North Americans to induce vomiting and for syphilis.
Medicinal discoveries Rhizome preparations have been investigated for cholesterol-lowering effects and antifungal and anti-inflammatory properties.

Isatis tinctoria
Woad

Originally found growing in the Caucasus. Biennial with small yellow flowers in the summer. Leaves turn dark green when growing in an alkaline soil.

Part(s) used Aerial parts, root.
Traditional uses Culpeper (see page 81) wrote that 'the root ointment is excellently good for such ulcers as abound with moisture, and takes away the corroding and fretting humours: it cools inflammations, quenches St Anthony's fire and stays defluxion of the blood to any part of the body.' Roots are used in traditional Chinese medicine to reduce fevers.
Medicinal discoveries Studies show it has antiviral and anti-inflammatory properties.

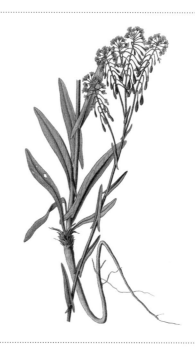

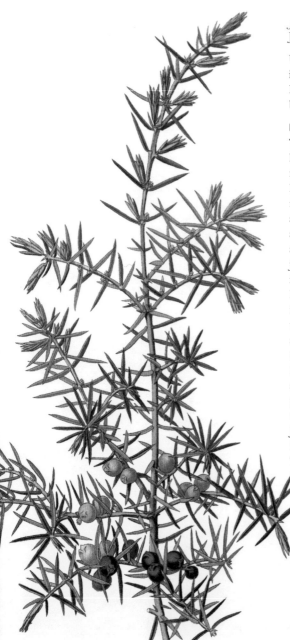

Juniperus communis
Juniper

Upright or spreading evergreen shrub that is widespread in the northern hemisphere. It produces green fruits (berries) that turn black-grey. Numerous cultivars.

Part(s) used Fruit.

Traditional uses Juniper oil was reputed to have diuretic properties and was taken as a remedy for kidney and bladder problems. It was also used for digestive complaints and flatulence. The oil was mixed with lard and applied to wounds in animals. Juniper was also used for dropsy and chest complaints and preparations were applied to alleviate joint pains. Native North Americans used it for dandruff and for syphilis. Juniper berries have been taken as a herbal medicine for indigestion (dyspepsia). The berries are also used in the manufacture of spirits and liqueurs.

Medicinal discoveries Scientific studies have revealed that juniper preparations and some berry constituents might have diuretic properties. However, there has been concern that juniper might irritate the kidneys. Juniper preparations also show anti-inflammatory and antimicrobial effects. The oil has been found to stimulate the uterus and juniper has been associated with antifertility effects. Juniper might also have effects on blood pressure. Studies are lacking to understand if these biological activities occur in humans.

Krameria lappacea
Rhatany

Perennial shrub from the Andes mountains with hairy, silver leaves and red flowers. It is hemiparasitic, ie, growing on the roots of other plants, and so difficult to cultivate.

Part(s) used Root.
Traditional uses Used to treat chronic diarrhoea, dysentery, abnormal periods, incontinence, blood in the urine and as a gargle to treat sore throat. Added to water to wash eyes, nose and gums. Still used as a mouthwash and can be found as an ingredient in toothpastes.
Medicinal discoveries Laboratory studies have shown that rhatany extracts have anti-inflammatory activity and can also inhibit the formation of biofilm (see p218).

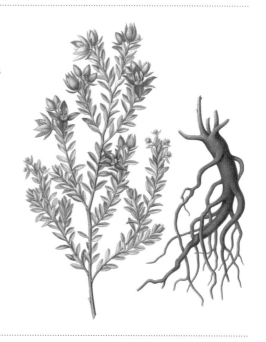

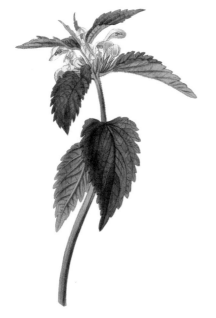

Lamium album
White nettle

Perennial herb from Europe and Asia with white flowers arranged around the axils on the square stem. Grows in moist fertile soils in most habitats.

Part(s) used Aerial parts.
Traditional uses Used for female health problems, especially thrush and the control of excess menstrual bleeding. Also taken as an anti-inflammatory for gastrointestinal problems, for wound healing and to control dandruff. Preparations of the flowers were used to treat gastrointestinal ailments.
Medicinal discoveries Laboratory studies have shown that the plant contains saponin and flavonoid compounds that contribute to its anti-inflammatory properties.

Lavandula angustifolia
English Lavender

René-Maurice Gattefossé was a French chemist who coined the phrase *aromathérapie*. In 1910, while carrying out research in his laboratory, he was caught in an explosion that covered him in burning substances. He quickly ran outside and rolled around on the grass. When his burnt hands later started to develop gas gangrene, he intuitively rinsed them in lavender essential oil. This prevented the spread and his burns healed faster than they had from previous accidents. Gattefossé went on to work with doctors in the First World War, treating French soldiers with essential oils. Lavender essential oil is now a common home remedy for minor burns, insect bites and wounds. Studies show it has a broad action against a range of infective microbes.

Botanist Richard Brook, in his book *A New Family Herbal* (published 1870) recommends lavender as 'good against all disorders of the head and nerves', reflecting the long-held reputation of lavender for calming worries and aiding sleep. The dried flowers hold their scent for a long time and make a refreshing tea suited to ease both digestive disturbances and headaches of nervous origin. Studies have shown inhaling the scent of lavender reduces alertness and memory, while improving general contentment.

Grow 'English' lavender is originally from the mountains of Spain, France and Italy. Enjoys well-drained neutral to alkaline soil in full sun. Flowers throughout summer.
Harvest Cut flowers at the base of stalks and hang up in bunches to dry. Rub flowers into a jar to store.

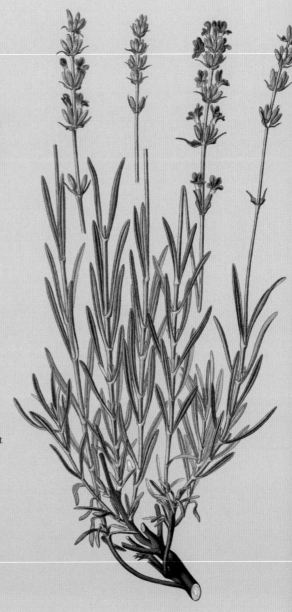

Lavender eye pillow

Place this lavender-filled pillow over your eyes
before bed or when you need a few moments to
relax. The soothing aroma will help you unwind.

30 x 10 cm (12 x 4 in) close-weave cotton fabric

3 tablespoons dried lavender flowers

150 g (5 oz) linseed

You will also need: sharp scissors; needle and
thread or dressmaker's pins; sewing machine;
scales; jug

1. To make the pillow, fold the fabric in half
lengthways. Baste or pin together along the
long side and along one short side. Leaving a
1 cm (½ in) seam allowance, machine stitch
the edges of the pillow together, leaving one
short side open. Turn right side out and iron.

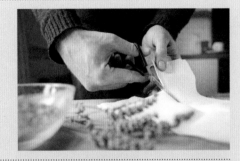

2. Mix the lavender and linseed together in
a jug, then pour into the pillow, filling it up
to two-thirds full.

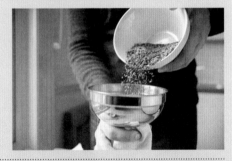

3. Fold the open edges of the bag inwards,
iron the seam, baste or pin in place, then
machine stitch closed.

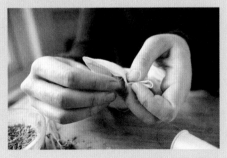

Leonurus cardiaca
Motherwort

Herbaceous perennial from Asia and Europe. Pink-lilac, hermaphrodite flowers appear in summer. A hedgerow plant, it is happiest in partial shade and in a well-drained soil.

Part(s) used Aerial parts.
Traditional uses Historically, motherwort was given for uterine infections and stress during pregnancy. In China it was used to prevent pregnancy and strengthen the heart.
Medicinal discoveries The plant contains the alkaloid leonurine which is thought to contribute to the ability of extracts to induce contractions of the uterus and for its cardiovascular uses. Clinical data are needed to support these claims.

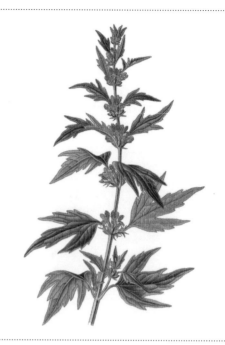

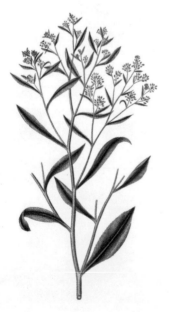

Lepidium latifolium
Pepperwort

Perennial from southern Europe and Asia, with waxy leaves and clusters of small, white flowers in early summer. An extensive root system can make it invasive. Dried stems are used in flower arrangements.

Part(s) used Aerial parts.
Traditional uses Used to treat stomach disorders as well as liver and kidney diseases. Reported to increase cardiac amplitude and regulate heart rhythms. It was used to treat skin disorders.
Medicinal discoveries There is very little known about the active ingredients in this plant.

Levisticum officinale
Lovage

Tall, aromatic, Mediterranean perennial with small, scented, green-yellow flowers and attractive leaves with a distinctive peppery, celery flavour.

Part(s) used Fruit, leaf, root.

Traditional uses In medieval times, lovage was associated with love potions and aphrodisiacs. The roots and fruit have been used for centuries as a remedy to aid digestion, reduce fevers and expel flatulence in children. The root was also used for menstrual and urinary disorders. The seventeenth-century herbalist Nicholas Culpeper (see page 81) claimed an infusion of the seeds 'dropped into the eyes taketh away their redness or dimness', that the herb decoction was 'effectual in pleurisy', and that preparations were 'good for quinsy if the mouth and throat be gargled'. Culpeper also claimed if the leaves were 'bruised and fried with a little hog's lard and laid hot to any blotch or boil will quickly break it'.

Medicinal discoveries Scientific studies have revealed that lovage root has antimicrobial and anti-inflammatory properties. It has been investigated for anticancer and diuretic effects. Root preparations also show oestrogen-like activities, which might explain the traditional use for menstrual disorders. Chemical components in the root appear to be able to suppress muscle spasms. There is interest in the use of the essential oil as an insect repellent.

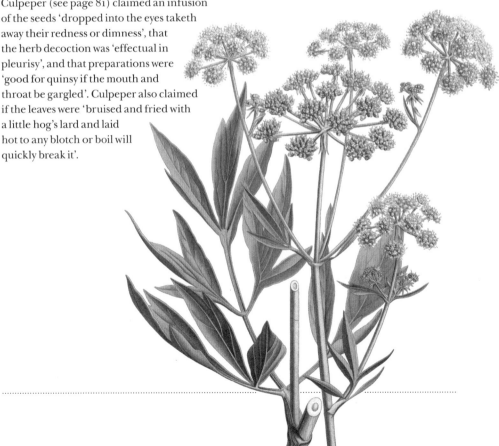

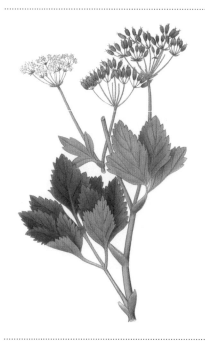

Ligusticum scoticum
Scots lovage, sea lovage

Clump-forming perennial from N. America and Europe; has been known to occur along Scottish coast. Produces green-white flowers in summer, followed by golden seed heads.

Part(s) used Leaf, root, stem.
Traditional uses The root was a remedy to aid digestion, improve circulation, and alleviate uterine disorders, rheumatic complaints and hysteria. The plant was boiled and eaten by sailors to combat scurvy. An infusion of the leaves was used as a purgative for calves.
Medicinal discoveries There are few scientific studies on *L. scoticum*. Chinese lovage (*L. sinense*) has been investigated as a potential treatment for obesity.

Ligustrum lucidum
Chinese privet

E. Asian and Chinese shrubby, evergreen tree with small, fragrant, cream-white flowers and glossy, dark green leaves.

Part(s) used Fruit.
Traditional uses A traditional Chinese medicine used as a liver and kidney tonic. It was also reputed to relieve menopausal symptoms and cure eye problems, such as blurred vision, and tinnitus. It was used to relieve aches and pains and aid sleep. Privet was also thought to combat greying hair.
Medicinal discoveries The fruit has been investigated for its potential to lower cholesterol. Scientific studies revealed the fruit might have anti-inflammatory, immune regulating and liver-protective properties.

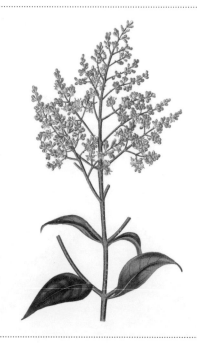

Linum usitatissimum
Flax, linseed

Native to the Mediterranean and central Asia, flax grows well in cool temperate regions. Although it's a commercial crop, it makes a pretty garden plant, too, with an abundance of bright blue flowers in summer.

Part(s) used Seed.

Traditional uses Used to treat a wide range of conditions including cardiovascular, respiratory and gastrointestinal disorders, eye infections, rheumatism, tumours and gout, and for controlling levels of cholesterol and blood sugar. Hot poultices were a popular remedy for treating boils and skin diseases such as eczema and herpes.

Medicinal discoveries Research suggests that the fatty acids and the lignan compounds in the seeds have potential as a treatment for cardiovascular conditions. Other studies have shown that flaxseed can influence the mobility and secretions in the gut: this could lead to the use of flax as a treatment for gastrointestinal disorders, especially diarrhoea. Flaxseed extracts also inhibit a range of pathogens associated with diarrhoea: a tea made from an infusion of the seeds mixed with honey and/or lime juice is considered a remedy for mild respiratory disorders and constipation. There is also interest in the use of the oil against breast and prostate cancers.

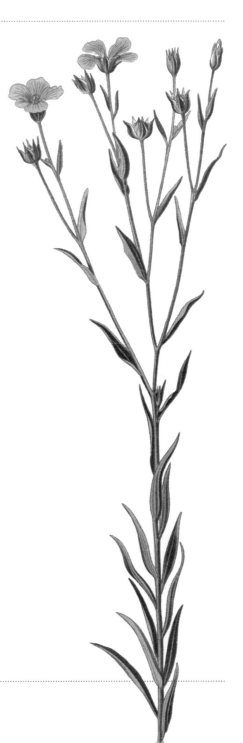

Lithospermum officinale
Common gromwell

European perennial found growing
in hedgerows and woodland borders.
It produces small green-white flowers
in summer followed by white nutlets.

Part(s) used Leaf, root, seed.
Traditional uses Mature seeds were used to
treat bladder stones, arthritis and febrile
conditions. Leaves were used as a sedative,
while roots were taken for smallpox, measles,
and kidney and bowel problems. Still used
by some herbalists as a tonic for kidney and
bowel disorders.
Medicinal discoveries Little is known about
the constituents in the plant that could
explain the traditional uses.

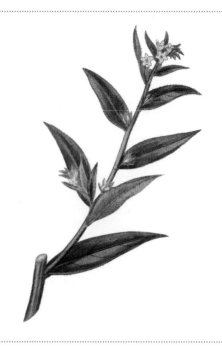

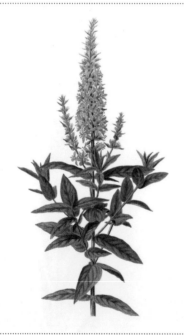

Lythrum salicaria
Purple loosestrife

Upright perennial with pink-purple flower
spikes in summer. Native to Europe, Asia
and N. Africa.

Part(s) used Aerial parts.
Traditional uses Reputed to have astringent
properties and was a traditional remedy
for diarrhoea, dysentery, blood-spitting,
fevers, sore throats, constipation, and liver
problems. It was applied to combat blindness
and soothe sore eyes, and used to clean and
heal wounds, sores and ulcers.
Medicinal discoveries Some scientific studies
suggest loosestrife has antidiarrhoeal,
antimicrobial and anti-inflammatory
properties. It has also been investigated for
effects on blood clotting.

Magnolia officinalis
Magnolia

Deciduous tree from western and central China now widely cultivated in temperate regions as an ornamental garden tree. The fragrant, cream-pink flowers appear in spring before the glossy green leaves. There are numerous species and cultivars.

Part(s) used Bark.

Traditional uses Used in traditional Chinese medicine, the bark was considered to have warming and relaxing properties. It was taken to aid digestion (the flowers were also made into a digestive tonic) and as a remedy for stomach pains, diarrhoea and vomiting, and for coughs and asthma. Other species of *Magnolia* were used by Native North Americans for fevers, rheumatic complaints and to prevent malaria: these include the cucumber tree (*M. acuminata*), umbrella tree (*M. tripetala*) and sweet bay (*M. virginiana*).

Medicinal discoveries Preparations of the bark and compounds isolated from the bark have been investigated for their potential to relieve anxiety. Preliminary studies have suggested some promising results, although more research is needed. Bark constituents have also been explored for their potential anticancer properties and for effects that might be relevant for use in Alzheimer's disease. The flowers have been investigated as a source of new anti-inflammatory and anti-allergic compounds.

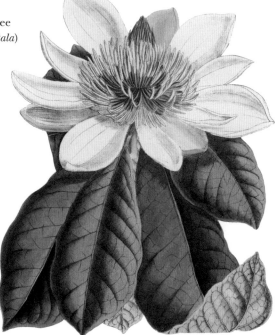

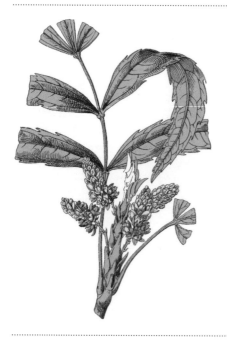

Mahonia fortunei
Chinese mahonia

A slow-growing, upright, evergreen shrub from China. Leaves are dark green on top and a pale yellowish green on the underside. Its sweet-scented, yellow flowers, which appear in winter, make this an attractive ornamental plant.

Part(s) used Leaf.
Traditional uses Used to treat eye infections, fevers, diarrhoea, indigestion, gout, rheumatic ailments, renal and bile diseases.
Medicinal discoveries Leaves contain the alkaloid berberine which has been shown to have a wide range of pharmacological properties that could in part explain some of the traditional uses.

Malus pumila
Crab apple

Tree that produces white-pink flowers in spring, followed by fruit that may vary in colour depending on the cultivar or variety.

Part(s) used Fruit.
Traditional uses Apples have a long history of use for health as the old rhyme 'an apple a day keeps the doctor away' suggests. Apples were considered to aid digestion, cure constipation and cleanse teeth. Rotten apples were applied as a poultice to sore eyes.
Medicinal discoveries Consumption of apples is suggested to reduce the risk of developing some cancers, heart disease and diabetes. Apples contain substances called tannins and those from *M. pumila* have been explored for potential benefits in arthritis.

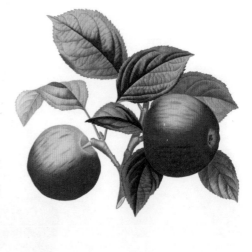

Malva neglecta
Common mallow

Sun-loving annual found growing in dry
soils in disturbed and waste ground in
Europe, N. Africa and Asia. Small, lilac-
white flowers appear in summer.

Part(s) used Aerial parts.
Traditional uses Taken for respiratory
diseases or inflammation of the digestive
or urinary systems. Used as a moisturizer,
diuretic, expectorant and laxative. A poultice
made from the leaves and flowers was used to
treat bruises, inflammation and insect bites.
Medicinal discoveries Laboratory studies
have shown that plant extracts have
anti-inflammatory properties that would
explain some of the traditional uses.

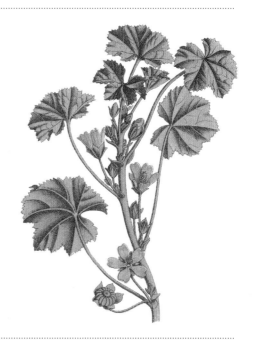

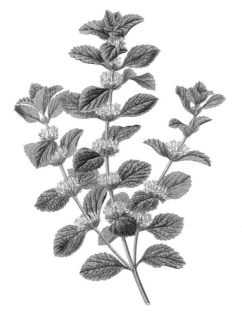

Marrubium vulgare
White horehound

Herbaceous perennial, native to Europe,
N. Africa and parts of Asia. White flowers
are produced over summer and autumn in
clusters on the upper part of the main stem.

Part(s) used Flower, leaf.
Traditional uses Used to aid digestion,
normalize heart rhythm, soothe sore
throats, ease coughs, bronchitis and
whooping cough and relieve inflammation.
Medicinal discoveries Shown to have
expectorant and vasodilative properties as
well as antimicrobial activity, which would
support some of its traditional uses. Plants
contain the compound marrubiin, which is
cardioactive and may protect against gastric
ulcers.

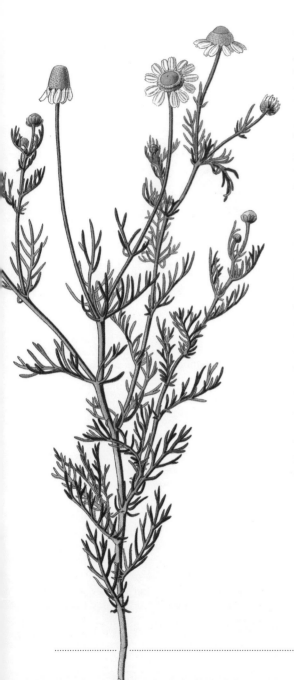

Matricaria chamomilla
German chamomile

Annual native to Europe and Asia with daisy-like, summer flowers that have a strong aromatic smell. Grows well along sunny paths in well-drained soils.

Part(s) used Flower.

Traditional uses Used to treat stomach and gastrointestinal problems including lack of appetite, colitis, diverticulitis, morning sickness and irritable bowel syndrome, as a gentle sleep aid and sedative, antiseptic, mild laxative and as an anti-inflammatory. It has also been used to treat asthma, dental problems, headaches, haemorrhoids, leg ulcers and wounds, and tired and sore eyes.

Medicinal discoveries Results from laboratory studies have supported many of the traditional uses, especially for its antibacterial, antifungal, antiviral, sedative and anti-inflammatory properties. These medicinal qualities are associated with compounds in the essential oil as well as the flavonoids extracted from the flower heads. There is also interest in the ability of chamomile extracts to regenerate liver tissue, lower blood cholesterol and for its use in ointments to improve wound healing in immune-compromised patients. More clinical data, however, are required to verify these various uses.

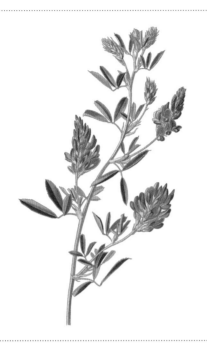

Medicago sativa
Lucerne, alfalfa

Perennial legume that can live from five to twenty years, thought to be originally from temperate parts of Asia. Resilient, drought-tolerant plant with a deep root system.

Part(s) used Aerial parts.
Traditional uses Medicinally used in the Americas and parts of Europe for treating heart and respiratory diseases and fluid retention, to regulate bowel movements, improve digestion and stimulate hair growth. Used by herbalists as a cardiotonic, emetic and for digestive disorders.
Medicinal discoveries Laboratory studies have shown the plant contains pharmacologically active compounds such as canavanine, isoflavones and saponins.

Melilotus officinalis
Melilot, yellow sweet clover

Aromatic, biennial herb with yellow honey-scented flowers. Occurs in Eurasia and North Africa. Once used as a strewing herb.

Part(s) used Aerial parts.
Traditional uses Used for the relief of pain and spasms and to treat varicose veins, sleep problems and flatulence. Melilot preparations were applied to draw out toxins and reduce swellings. Also made into a rat poison.
Medicinal discoveries Preparations are anti-inflammatory and might reduce fluid retention. They have been investigated for use in vein problems. The plant contains components which prevent blood clotting, and which could affect the liver. Use of the plant may cause side effects.

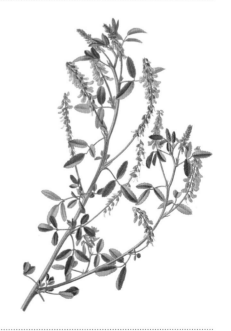

Melissa officinalis
Lemon balm

Ibn Sina (known as Avicenna), a Persian scholar and physician born in the late tenth century, wrote 'balm causeth the heart and mind to become merry', and recommended it to treat epilepsy. It has been used ever since for treating symptoms of stress, to aid sleep and for promoting memory; effects that have all been supported by clinical trials. The essential oil binds to receptors in the brain that are linked to reducing anxiety. Scientists at Kew collaborated with research teams at several universities to investigate the effect lemon balm lotion had on dementia sufferers. Although it did not significantly reduce symptoms of agitation, compared to a lotion without lemon balm, it did improve measures of quality of life and indicates possibilities for further research.

The Latin for balm, *balsam*, means a healing, aromatic extract. In the fourteenth century, Carmelite nuns developed an extract of lemon balm, nutmeg, coriander and angelica, known as Carmelite water, which was famed for its sweet scent and healing properties. There are myriad variations on this combination of lemon balm and other aromatic herbs in alcohol (often white wine).

Lemon balm is also used today for cold sores; studies have shown it is active against the virus that causes them.

Grow Needs a sheltered site in full sun in a well-drained soil. Flowers mid to late summer.
Harvest Pick leaves before flowering on a sunny day when the plant's essential oil content is at its highest. Harvest leaves from the top 10 cm (4 inch) of the plant.

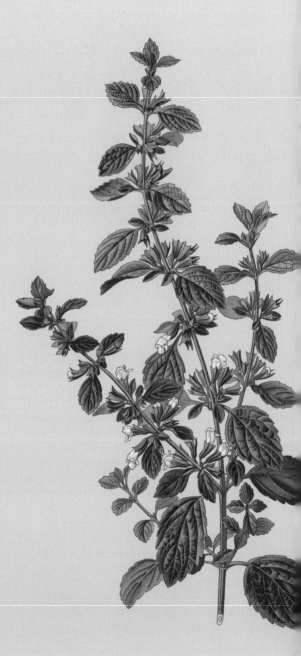

Dried lemon balm

This drying method can be used for all leaves and flowers. For the highest essential oil content, pick leaves before the plant has started to flower, and pick on a sunny afternoon when it will be producing the most essential oils. Use dried lemon balm to make tea – on its own or blended (see page 141) – and in tinctures.

Fresh lemon balm leaves

You will also need: a container, such as a basket, grocery crate or cardboard box; small brown paper bags; airtight plastic container or glass storage jar

1. Spread leaves in a single layer in a clean, dry container that will allow free circulation of air, such as a woven basket, a grocery crate or a cardboard box with lots of holes punched in the sides and bottom flaps.

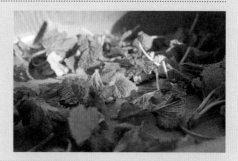

2. Leave the container in a warm, dry place away from direct sun. Raise up the container to improve the flow of air underneath. Turn leaves once a day until completely dry.

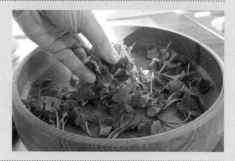

3. For maximum shelf life, store leaves in small brown paper bags in an airtight plastic container. Alternatively, store in a glass jar in a cool, dark place. Can keep for several years if dried and stored correctly, though the aroma will dissipate.

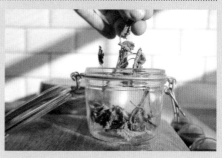

Mentha x piperita
Peppermint

Fragrant, upright, hardy perennial herb that is a hybrid of *Mentha aquatica* (watermint) and *M. spicata* (spearmint). Native of Europe. Leaves have a minty aroma with lilac-pink flowers. Mint plants come in many different forms, with various leaf tones and aromas.

Part(s) used Aerial parts.

Traditional uses In Greek mythology, the nymph Minthe was turned into a plant by the jealous queen Persephone. The word 'mint' can be traced back to this legend. The herb was used by the ancient Egyptians and it was described in thirteenth-century medicinal texts in Iceland. It was used more widely in Europe in the mid 18th century and was considered as a remedy for colic, flatulence and indigestion. It was reputed to alleviate diarrhoea, nausea and sickness and was used for cholera. It was also a remedy for nervous disorders, heart palpitations and hysteria.

Medicinal discoveries Peppermint oil capsules are an over-the-counter medicine to relieve irritable bowel syndrome. A main component of the essential oil from peppermint is a compound called menthol: this is included in some over-the-counter inhalation preparations to relieve nasal congestion; it is also included in creams and ointments to relieve itching.

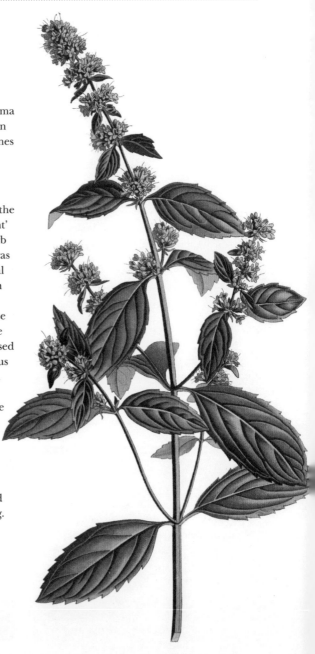

Mentha spicata
Spearmint, English lamb mint

Vigorous, aromatic, perennial herb from
Europe with pale pink, lilac or white flowers.
Unfussy about aspect and soil type, although
moist but well drained suits it best.

Part(s) used Leaf.
Traditional uses The herbalist John Gerard
(see page 81) claimed 'it is good against
watering eyes and all manner of breakings
out on the head and sores'. Spearmint was
also used to boost memory, as a gargle for
sore mouths and to soothe chapped hands.
Medicinal discoveries The essential oil from
the leaves has antibacterial and antifungal
properties. Spearmint tea has been
investigated for its potential to relieve
knee-joint pain.

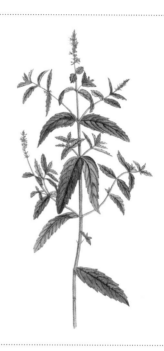

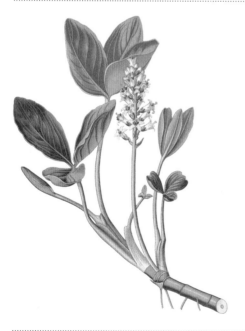

Menyanthes trifoliata
Bogbean

Aquatic, rhizomatous perennial found in
bogs in temperate areas across the northern
hemisphere. Green leaves form floating
mats; erect pale pink flowers in summer.

Part(s) used Leaf.
Traditional uses Used as tonic to treat fevers,
rheumatism, scurvy, gout and skin diseases.
Leaves are reported to have carminative,
anti-inflammatory, digestive, emetic and
diuretic properties. Given to people who
needed to gain weight and strength after
viral infections. Used by herbalists to treat
rheumatoid arthritis and as a general tonic.
Medicinal discoveries Laboratory studies
have shown that extracts of the plant have
antioxidant and antibacterial properties.

Mitchella repens
Partridge berry

Evergreen, woody shrub with dark shiny leaves and small, white trumpet-shaped flowers. Originally from N. America and Mexico. A good rockery plant or for growing in the shade under trees.

Part(s) used Fruit, leaf.
Traditional uses Native North American women made a tea from the leaves and fruits to relieve urinary problems and to decrease pain during childbirth. Also used in early pregnancy to prevent miscarriage.
Medicinal discoveries Laboratory studies have shown that extracts of the plant have antibacterial properties that could explain its traditional use in treating urinary infections.

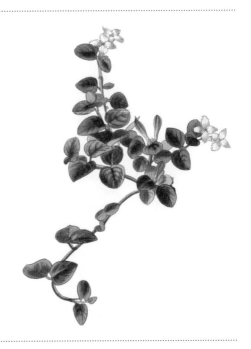

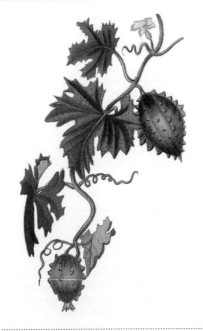

Momordica charantia
Balsam pear, bitter cucumber

Climbing annual and perennial from tropical and subtropical Africa and Asia. It produces yellow flowers and warty gourds.

Part(s) used Fruit, leaf.
Traditional uses Widely used as a remedy for diabetes. Leaves were used for intestinal worms and fevers. Skin problems, including burns, were treated topically with fruit preparations.
Medicinal discoveries There has been much interest in the potential use of the fruit in controlling diabetes. Scientific studies revealed that components of the fruits and the leaves can reduce blood glucose levels; however, when tested in people with type 2 diabetes, there was insufficient evidence they had any effect on glucose control.

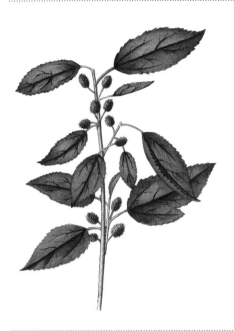

Morus alba
White mulberry

Deciduous tree from China with edible, white fruits that turn red-purple as they ripen.

Part(s) used Leaf, root bark, twig.
Traditional uses In traditional Chinese medicine, leaves and root bark (stripped from the root and dried) were used as a diuretic and to alleviate inflammatory disorders. Fruits were believed to aid sleep and young branches were used to treat joint and rheumatic complaints.
Medicinal discoveries Different plant parts have been investigated in many scientific studies, although there is a lack of clinical studies. Mulberry has been of interest for potential antidiabetic and cholesterol-lowering properties.

Mucuna pruriens
Velvet bean

Annual climber with deep purple, lilac or white flowers. Occurs in parts of Asia, although naturalized elsewhere.

Part(s) used Seed.
Traditional uses Used for male infertility, as an aphrodisiac and to treat nervous disorders. In traditional Indian medicine, particularly in Ayurvedic, it was used for controlling diabetes and the symptoms of Parkinson's disease.
Medicinal discoveries Bean extracts have been investigated for their potential to alleviate symptoms of Parkinson's disease. Velvet beans contain levodopa, the same type of chemical that is used as a drug to treat Parkinson's disease symptoms.

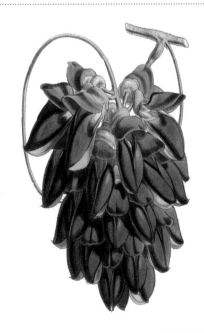

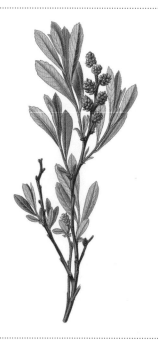

Myrica gale
Sweet gale

Deciduous, bushy shrub native to peaty areas in Europe and N. America. The willow-like, dark green leaves are fragrant when bruised. Flowers are known as catkins.

Part(s) used Leaf.
Traditional uses In Europe, America and China, leaves were used in infusions to treat stomach ache, fever and bronchial and liver problems. Leaves were made into a cordial to relieve extreme thirst and added to ointments to treat skin conditions.
Medicinal discoveries Laboratory experiments have supported the use of the essential oil as a repellent for the highland midge. It has also been shown to have mild antibacterial properties.

Myristica fragrans
Nutmeg

Small evergreen tree indigenous to the Indonesian Spice Islands. The flowers are bell-shaped and pale yellow; the fruit is yellow with red and green markings. The seed (nutmeg) is covered with a red membrane (mace).

Part(s) used Seed.
Traditional uses The essential oil from the nutmeg was taken for disorders related to the nervous and digestive systems. Also added to toothpastes and cough medicines.
Medicinal discoveries Laboratory tests have shown that the essential oil has anti-inflammatory, antiviral and antibacterial properties and can be hallucinogenic. It should be used in small amounts.

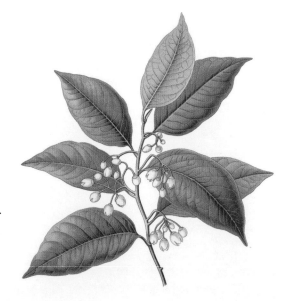

Myroxylon balsamum
Tolu balsam

Tall tree from Central America with small white flowers and winged seed pods. An aromatic resin is harvested from the tree by cutting into the bark and collecting the sap.

Part(s) used Resin.
Traditional uses The aromatic resin was used as a treatment for haemorrhoids, tuberculosis, venereal diseases, coughs, asthma, bronchitis, headaches, colds and flu, rheumatism, wounds and skin problems. It was added to lozenges to treat coughs and sore throats.
Medicinal discoveries Laboratory studies have shown it can stop bacterial biofilms forming; which could explain some of its traditional uses.

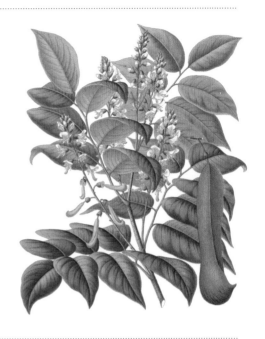

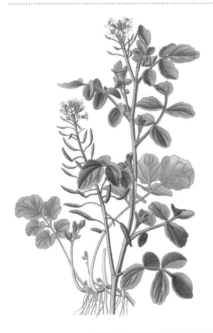

Nasturtium officinale
Watercress

Pungent perennial herb with white flowers from Europe and northern Asia. Needs full sun, prefers wet soil and can grow in water.

Part(s) used Aerial parts.
Traditional uses Taken as a digestive aid and to improve appetite, as a remedy for coughs, catarrhs and mouth inflammations. The plant had a reputation for purifying the blood and was considered a 'spring cure'.
Medicinal discoveries Watercress contains antioxidant constituents, including beta-carotene, which help protect cells in the body from damage. There has also been interest in its potential anticancer effects. Herb preparations have anti-inflammatory and antibacterial properties.

Nepeta cataria
Catnip, catmint

Herbaceous perennial found in temperate areas in Europe. From spring to autumn it produces small, white, fragrant flowers spotted with pink or purple.

Part(s) used Aerial parts.
Traditional uses An infusion of catnip was given for fevers, to promote sleep, soothe stomach problems and as a carminative. It was made into a poultice to reduce painful swellings. Combined with saffron it was considered a cure for scarlet fever and smallpox. Catnip is still used as an infusion for early signs of a cold or upset stomach.
Medicinal discoveries The plant contains a range of compounds that have antiviral and antibacterial properties.

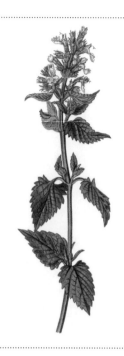

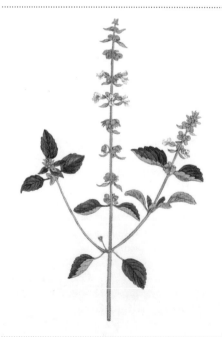

Ocimum basilicum
Basil

Frost-tender, aromatic annual from tropical Africa and Asia, now widely grown as a commercial crop. Cultivars offer a range of subtle flavours (hints of lemon, clove, anise), leaf colour (from green to deep purple), and flower colour (white to magenta). The plant needs full sun and rich, well-drained soil.

Part(s) used Aerial parts.
Traditional uses Used to treat inflammatory conditions, skin disorders, cardiac diseases, gynaecological disorders, respiratory problems including asthma and whooping cough, fevers and diabetes.
Medicinal discoveries Essential oil has anti-inflammatory properties; water extracts have antibacterial and antiviral activity.

Ocimum tenuiflorum
Holy basil, tulsi

Frost-tender, sun-loving annual, native
to the Indian subcontinent where it is
considered a sacred plant. There are two
cultivated forms, one with green leaves, the
other with purple. Both produce purple
flowers from spring to late autumn. Will
grow in a wide range of soils. This plant is
often known as *Ocimum sanctum*.

Part(s) used Aerial parts.

Traditional uses Used for thousands of years
in Ayurvedic medicine as an adaptogen: a
herbal remedy used to balance different
processes in the body. It is regarded as an
elixir of life and taken to promote longevity.
Possesses a broad range of reported activity
as an analgesic, antifertility, anticancer,
antidiabetic, antifungal and antimicrobial.
It also offers protective properties for liver
and heart. It was used externally to treat
wounds and skin conditions. The essential
oils were used to repel insects. It is still used
in Ayurvedic medicine for a wide range
of conditions.

Medicinal discoveries Essential oil from
the leaves contains many biologically
active compounds, including eugenol and
caryophyllene, that show anti-inflammatory
and antioxidant properties that account
for some of the traditional uses of the
plant. Other studies show that polyphenol
compounds in the leaves could explain how
the plant regulates gene expression when
used for heart conditions and diabetes.

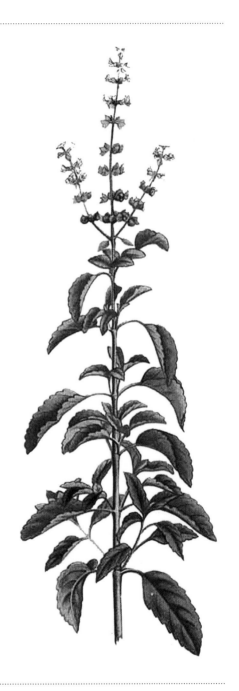

Oenothera biennis
Evening primrose

A biennial with fragrant, bright yellow flowers that open in the evening. From N. America but widely naturalized elsewhere.

Part(s) used Whole plant, seed oil.

Traditional uses Preparations of the whole plant or the leaves were considered to aid sleep and relieve pain, asthma, coughs and gastrointestinal problems. Leaves were a remedy for 'female complaints' and for regulating menstruation. Traditionally, poultices were applied to aid healing of wounds and bruises.

Medicinal discoveries The seed oil contains fatty acids, particularly gamma-linolenic acid (GLA). There has been much interest in the use of the oil for a range of health problems, in particular eczema and premenstrual syndrome. Although some studies show promising effects, more evidence is needed to support these uses of evening primrose oil. The oil has also been investigated for potential use in multiple sclerosis and in nerve damage that can occur in diabetes. Other possible uses have been explored and include for rheumatoid arthritis, heart disease and dementia. The oil is also widely used in skin preparations for cosmetic use.

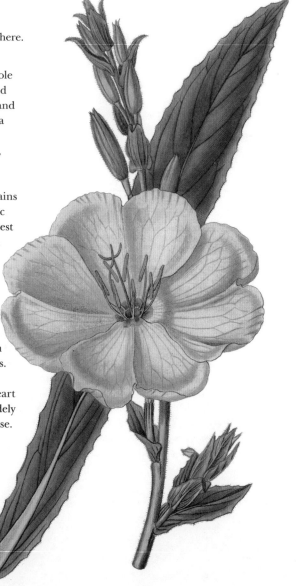

Olea europaea
Olive

Evergreen tree, generally long-lived, originating from the Mediterranean region.

Part(s) used Fruit oil, leaf.
Traditional uses Leaves were used as a diuretic and for high blood pressure. They were considered to have calming properties, to ease nervous tension and were applied for skin problems and cuts.
Medicinal discoveries Olive oil has been used to soothe sore throats, as a laxative, and is applied to soothe inflamed skin. It is an ingredient of some medicinal ointments and suspensions and is used to soften earwax. The oil has also been of interest in the prevention of heart disease and has been investigated for effects against cancer.

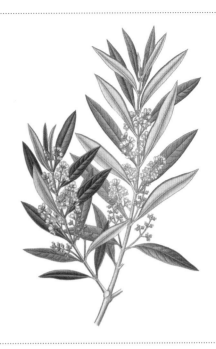

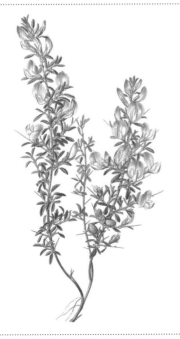

Ononis spinosa
Spiny restharrow

Small perennial shrub native to Europe and N. Africa with spiny thorns on the stems. Pink-purple blooms in summer. Grows on chalk, limestone and calcareous clay soils.

Part(s) used Aerial parts, root.
Traditional uses Traditionally used for bladder stones and to subdue delirium. Also used as a diuretic in cardiac-related conditions, as a mild antiseptic and to treat gout, inflammation of the kidneys and bladder, and rheumatism.
Medicinal discoveries Scientific studies have shown it has anti-inflammatory properties which could explain its use for inflammatory ailments.

Ophiopogon japonicus
Mondo grass, lily turf

Evergreen perennial originally from eastern Asia. Useful ground-cover plant with dark green, narrow leaves and white flowers in late summer followed by blue berries.

Part(s) used Tuber.

Traditional uses Traditional Chinese medicine reputed to have soothing and sedative properties, it was used for insomnia and anxiety. Also taken as a remedy for coughs as it was believed to lubricate the airways and the digestive system. Other traditional uses were for treating constipation, thirst and fevers.

Medicinal discoveries Anti-inflammatory and anti-blood clotting properties found in laboratory studies. Clinical trials needed.

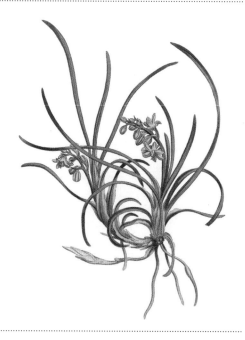

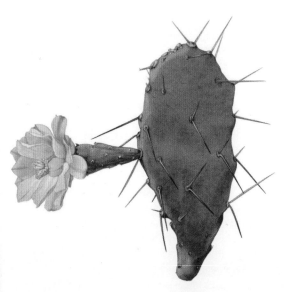

Opuntia ficus-indica
Prickly pear, Indian fig

Prickly cactus originally from Mexico. White, red or yellow flowers appear in early summer followed by edible purple fruits.

Part(s) used Fruit.

Traditional uses Used to treat diabetes, obesity, colitis, diarrhoea, benign prostatic hypertrophy (enlarged prostate gland) and to make a tonic to fight viral infections.

Medicinal discoveries Scientific research has shown that extracts of the fruit can lower blood glucose and also inhibit the expression of genes involved in inflammatory responses. Some health drinks contain fruit extracts because they have been shown to have antioxidant properties.

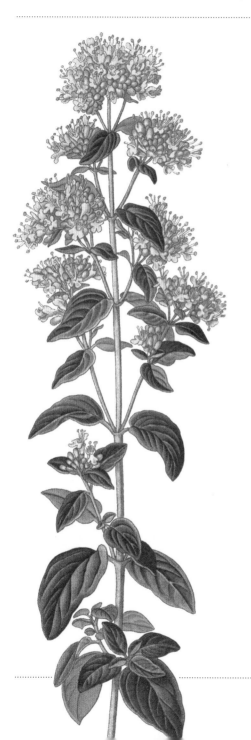

Origanum vulgare
Oregano, wild marjoram

A highly aromatic, bushy perennial from S.W. Asia and the Mediterranean with dark green leaves and pink-white flowers in late summer. Popular culinary herb; different cultivars available.

Part(s) used Flower, leaf.
Traditional uses Used to treat digestive problems, mouth and throat infections, fevers, cuts and wounds, and to soothe bites and stings. It was reputed to stimulate the uterus and relieve menstrual pain, and, when applied to the skin, to relieve joint and muscle pains. In the Ancient Greek text *Enquiry into Plants*, written by Theophrastus, *Origanum dictamnus* (known as Cretan dittany) was described as 'marvellous in virtue and is useful for many purposes, but especially for women in childbirth'.
Medicinal discoveries The essential oil from oregano contains a compound called thymol, which has antiseptic properties. Most scientific studies on oregano have focused on its antimicrobial properties and the oil has shown activity against a range of bacteria and fungi. The oil has also been investigated for its effects on cancer cells; other constituents of the plant have been of interest for use in diabetes. Preparations of the plant show antioxidant effects and have been explored for their potential to help protect the liver.

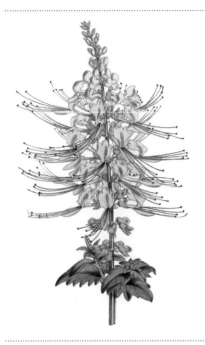

Orthosiphon aristatus
Java tea, cat's whiskers

Shrub from N.E. Australia that produces white or lilac flowers.

Part(s) used Leaf, stem.
Traditional uses Known as a remedy for rheumatic complaints, bladder and kidney disorders, and for its diuretic action. In Java it was taken for high blood pressure and diabetes.
Medicinal discoveries Modern interest in Java tea has focused on its diuretic properties, with promising effects in some studies, although more research is needed. Other studies suggest the plant and its constituents might lower blood glucose and blood pressure levels. Preparations also have antimicrobial properties.

Oxalis acetosella
Wood sorrel

Creeping, mat-forming perennial native to Europe. Small rose-pink blooms appear in spring to midsummer. At night or when raining the flowers close and leaves fold. Grows in full shade making it a useful ground-cover plant under trees or shrubs.

Part(s) used Leaf.
Traditional uses Used as a diuretic and expectorant, to treat fevers and stomach aches. A poultice was made of crushed leaves and applied to wounds, boils and abscesses.
Medicinal discoveries Scientific studies have shown that the leaves contain oxalic acid which can cause the precipitation of calcium oxalate associated with kidney stones and some joint pain – should be used with caution.

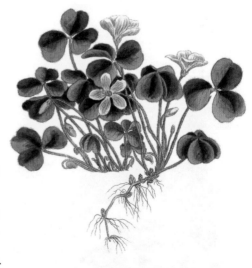

Paeonia lactiflora
Chinese peony

Herbaceous perennial native to eastern
and western Asia. Fragrant, white to pale
pink flowers with yellow stamens produced
in early summer. Many cultivars available.

Part(s) used Root.
Traditional uses Used as a diuretic and for
treating flatulence, nosebleeds, wounds and
other haemorrhages as well as fevers, colds,
nervous disorders, headaches and menstrual
difficulties. Used in traditional Chinese
medicine to treat menstrual pain, sweating,
headaches and chest and stomach pains.
Medicinal discoveries Laboratory tests have
shown extracts can modulate muscle spasm,
relieve pain and improve blood circulation.

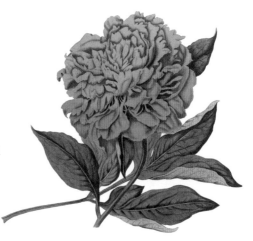

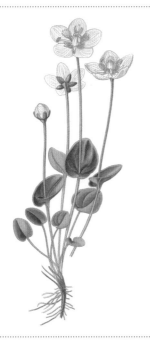

Parnassia palustris
Grass of Parnassus

Small hardy perennial native to Europe
found in wet, boggy soils. In summer it
produces delicate, single, white-green flowers
with yellow stamens on long, thin stems.

Part(s) used Flowering aerial parts.
Traditional uses The plant is astringent and
was used to treat wounds, as a mild diuretic, as
a sedative, for treating nervous disorders and
epileptic fits. Decoctions were used as an eye
lotion and a mouthwash. It is used as a
homeopathic tonic for anxiety.
Medicinal discoveries Very little is known
about the chemistry of this plant.

Passiflora incarnata
Passionflower

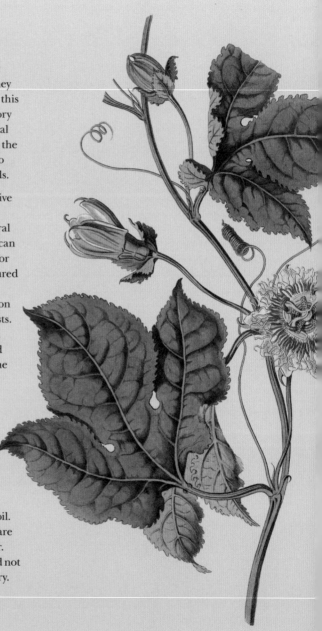

The first Europeans to come across the passionflower were the Spanish Catholic soldiers who invaded South America. They named it passiflora because each part of this unusual flower reminded them of the story of Christ's passion: for example, the radial filaments represent the crown of thorns, the three stigma the nails that hung Christ to the cross, and the five anthers the wounds.

Seeds of *Passiflora incarnata*, which is native to eastern North America, have been found on sites of human habitation several thousand years old. Native North American Cherokees used the root in an infusion for treating boils, to wean children, and poured into the ear for earache. The pounded root was applied to draw out inflammation from wounds caused by thorns and locusts. Infusions of leaves were used for anxiety. Passionflower fruits were enjoyed as food and to make drinks. (*Passiflora edulis* is the species more favoured for its fruit.)

Studies have shown that in combination with other herbs, such as hops and valerian, *P. incarnata* can help improve sleep quality. Herbalists also use it for Parkinson's disease and shingles pain.

Grow Hardy, evergreen climber that will quickly grow to 6 m (20 ft). Flowers in summer. Needs sun and prefers a moist soil.
Harvest Both the leaves and the flowers are used and can be picked over the summer.
Caution Can cause drowsiness and should not be taken if driving or operating machinery.

Passionflower sleep tea

Herbal teas brewed for medicinal purposes tend to be stronger than those made for their flavour. If the taste is too bitter, add a little liquorice to the brew or stir in some honey. Drink a cup before bedtime.

3 tablespoons dried passionflowers

1 tablespoon dried valerian root

2 tablespoons dried lemon balm leaves

½ tablespoon dried lavender flowers

500 ml (17 fl oz) boiling water

½ teaspoon liquorice or honey, optional sweetners

You will also need: teapot; tablespoon; teaspoon; tea strainer; measuring jug

1. Herbal teas or tisanes are best brewed in a teapot; it is less messy, increases the extraction and prevents volatile oils escaping. Warm the pot first, if you like, then add the dried herbs. If you like a little sweetness, add half a teaspoon of dried liquorice to the brew.

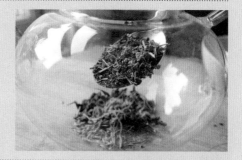

2. Pour over freshly boiled water and leave to steep for ten to fifteen minutes.

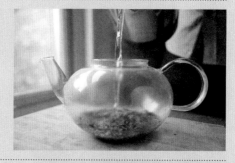

3. Pour out using a strainer. If you need further sweetening, stir in honey to taste. Any leftover tea can be kept in the fridge for up to three days and reheated as required.

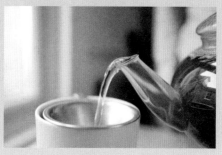

Pelargonium reniforme
Pelargonium, sweetheart geranium

Perennial originally from S. Africa; in colder climates it is grown as an annual. Produces white, pink, lilac or purple flowers.

Part(s) used Root.
Traditional uses Given as a treatment for respiratory infections, for tuberculosis, dysentery, diarrhoea, liver problems and menstrual disorders. Preparations were applied to the skin to heal wounds.
Medicinal discoveries The plant's efficacy as a remedy for respiratory infections is the subject of current scientific interest. Studies suggest roots and their constituents have antibacterial and antiviral properties and that they may aid the immune response.

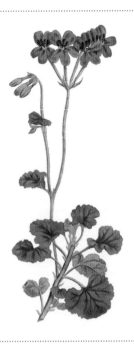

Perilla frutescens
Beefsteak plant

Leafy annual with white flowers in summer followed by small brown nutlets. Originally from Asia and naturalized in N. America.

Part(s) used Leaf, seed, stem.
Traditional uses Traditional Chinese medicine valued for its warming and expectorant properties. Seeds were thought to alleviate colds and chills, nausea, spasms, digestive complaints and respiratory disorders, such as asthma and bronchitis. Stems were given for morning sickness.
Medicinal discoveries Grown as a food plant and as an ornamental. It has been investigated for anti-allergic, anti-inflammatory and anticancer properties. Possible potential for it to alleviate hay fever.

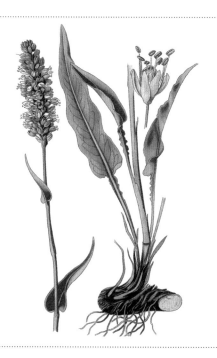

Persicaria bistorta
Bistort, adderwort

Perennial from northern Europe and Asia that produces spikes of pink flowers.

Part(s) used Rhizome, root.
Traditional uses Used as a soothing remedy to promote healing and treat symptoms of diarrhoea, dysentery and cholera. Preparations were taken for menstrual problems and were applied to wounds, haemorrhoids and to snake and insect bites.
Medicinal discoveries Scientific studies suggest some root constituents have anti-inflammatory properties. Root p reparations have been investigated for protective effects on blood vessels and for anticancer effects.

Petroselinum crispum
Parsley

Bright green, biennial native to central and southern Europe. Grows best in moist, well-drained soil in full sun. Has small yellow-green flowers. Can be grown in pots or cultivated beds.

Part(s) used Leaf, root (second year old).
Traditional uses Used as a diuretic to treat gout, jaundice, rheumatism and remove 'gravel and stones' from the kidneys. Parsley tea was given to soldiers in the First World War for dysentery.
Medicinal discoveries Scientific experiments have shown that root extracts can decrease uric acid content, which could explain why it was used for treating gout.

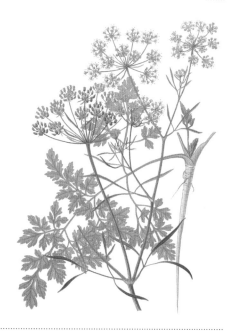

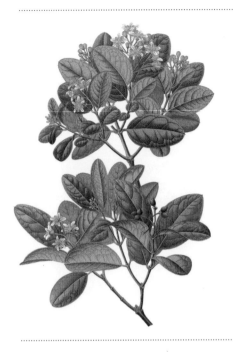

Peumus boldus
Boldo

Evergreen shrub, or small tree, which occurs in Chile. Produces aromatic leaves and fragrant clusters of flowers.

Part(s) used Leaf.
Traditional uses In South America, boldo was used to treat gonorrhoea. The leaves were reputed to have tonic and stimulant properties and were taken for liver disorders, as a diuretic and for urinary infections. Leaves were taken to expel intestinal worms.
Medicinal discoveries Boldo has been of interest for digestive complaints. Laboratory studies have revealed that it might have liver-protective and anti-inflammatory properties. The essential oil is considered to be irritant and toxic.

Phaseolus vulgaris
Common bean

Herbaceous annual native to the Americas. Cultivars come in climbing, trailing, erect and bushy forms with white, pink, or purple flowers followed by pods of edible beans.

Part(s) used Aerial parts.
Traditional uses Considered a remedy for acne, diabetes, diarrhoea, coughs, eczema, rheumatism, arthritis and hiccups. Ground seeds were used to make a flour that was applied to ulcers. A homeopathic remedy is made from the aerial parts of the fresh herb for rheumatism and arthritis, plus disorders of the urinary tract.
Medicinal discoveries Most research is focused on the nutritional properties of *P. vulgaris* rather than its medicinal uses.

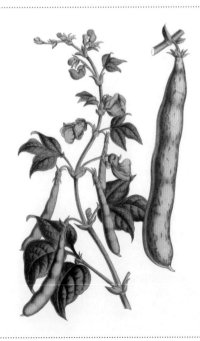

Phlebodium aureum
Golden polypody, hare's foot fern

An evergreen fern occurring in Central and South America, the West Indies and parts of Southeast USA. Makes a good pot plant; needs protection from frost.

Part(s) used Aerial parts, rhizome.
Traditional uses Leaves were used to treat kidney problems, stomach ulcers and joint pains. Also considered a remedy for skin disorders such as psoriasis. The rhizome is a traditional remedy for cough and cold symptoms, liver disorders and constipation.
Medicinal discoveries Research has focused on its use for treating skin problems, such as vitiligo, psoriasis and inflamed skin. It might also help protect the skin from UV radiation.

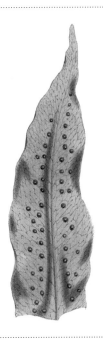

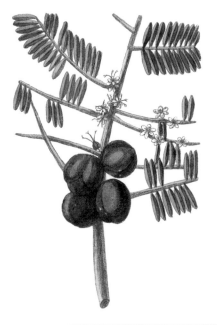

Phyllanthus emblica
Indian gooseberry, amla

Small- to medium-sized tree native to Asia and parts of Australia. Will grow in warm dry areas. Has light green leaves and green-yellow flowers followed by spherical, pale green fruits, called gooseberries.

Part(s) used Fruit, but all parts used.
Traditional uses Used in traditional Indian and Chinese medicine to promote longevity, improve digestion, treat eye problems, constipation, cough, asthma, fevers and heart problems.
Medicinal discoveries Scientific research has shown it has antiviral and antimicrobial properties and modulates the expression of cells involved in rheumatoid arthritis and osteoporosis.

Pimpinella anisum
Anise

Frost-tender, aromatic annual, native to
N.E. Africa. Needs sun and well-drained but
moist soil. Green feathery leaves with white
summer flowers produced in dense umbels.
Seeds are familiarly known as anise.

Part(s) used Seed pod.
Traditional uses Used to treat flatulence,
coughs, especially dry coughs, and for
clearing the bronchial tubes in cases of
bronchitis and asthma. It is still used in
lozenges for coughs.
Medicinal discoveries Preliminary scientific
research has shown that anise can reduce
cell damage caused by the breakdown of
lipids. This could be a significant finding in
the treatment of diabetes.

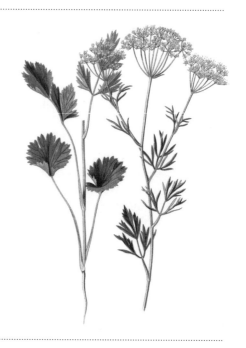

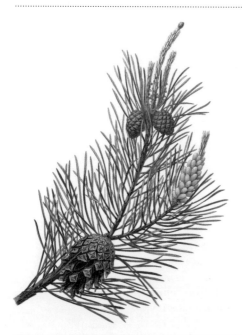

Pinus sylvestris
Scots pine

Evergreen, coniferous tree, native to Eurasia.
Tall, straight trunk with orange-red bark
topped by a rounded mass of blue-green
needle-like leaves. Green female cones ripen
to grey or red-brown.

Part(s) used Leaf resin.
Traditional uses Essential oil extracted from
the leaves was used as an antiseptic and for
respiratory and digestive ailments. Resin
was used as a remedy for kidney, bladder and
rheumatic disorders. Essential oil is used
in aromatherapy and added to products
for relieving chest infections and to bath
products to combat stress and fatigue.
Medicinal discoveries Resin contains many
compounds with medicinal properties.

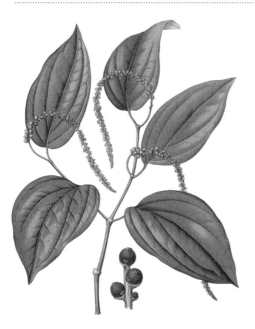

Piper nigrum
Black pepper

Perennial woody vine native to S.E. Asia. Grows well in moist, well-drained and organically rich soils. Plants bear fruit from the fourth or fifth year and continue doing so for seven years.

Part(s) used Pod, seed.
Traditional uses Given as a treatment for fevers, urinary and gastrointestinal disorders and as a stimulant.
Medicinal discoveries The main biologically active compound in pepper is the alkaloid piperine. In scientific studies, pepper and piperine have been shown to modulate receptors in the gut, which could explain the use of pepper in gastrointestinal disorders.

Pistacia lentiscus
Mastic tree

Evergreen shrub or small tree found in Mediterranean Europe in scrubby, rocky areas by the sea. It has small red flowers and red fruits ripening to black. Mastic is collected from cuts made in the tree bark.

Part(s) used Bark resin (mastic).
Traditional uses The mastic tree has a long history of use in the treatment of gastrointestinal ailments. Also used in ointments to treat skin disorders and chewed to reduce mouth infections.
Medicinal discoveries Research has shown that the resin has antibacterial properties and when chewed can reduce plaque in the mouth. The antibacterial properties could explain its use in skin remedies.

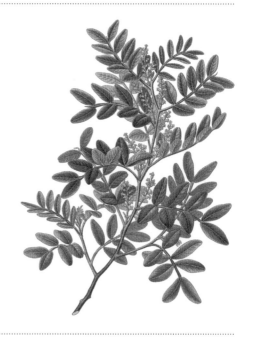

Plantago lanceolata
Ribwort plantain

Ribwort plantain and its close relative greater plantain (*Plantago major*) were introduced to N. America by European colonizers. The Native Americans called them white man's footsteps as they grew along footpaths on grasslands. The name *Plantago* comes from *planta* (foot).

The plant's adaptability and quick growth means they are often dismissed as a weed, but they were once highly valued as medicine. The *Lacnuga*, a tenth- to eleventh-century collection of Anglo-Saxon medicine and prayers, includes plantain in the 'Nine herbs charm'. This was both a recipe for a salve and an incantation, which were used together to treat poison and 'flying venom'. Plantain was said to withstand this affliction in the same way it withstood the trampling of bulls and chariots.

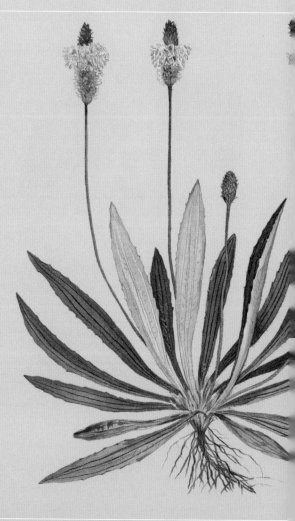

Both plantain species are still used in traditional medicine for treating wounds and burns, and as a poultice or salve for drawing out splinters. Freshly picked leaves of plantain are used to treat insect stings and bites, as well as nettle rash. The apparent anti-allergic action is the basis for their use for inflamed sinuses and hayfever, taken as a tea or tincture. In Eastern Europe a syrup of ribwort plantain is available as a remedy for coughs and colds. A less common use is to help heal the lining of the digestive tract.

Grow Perennial ribwort plantain is found in lawns and will tolerate regular mowing.
Harvest Leaves can be picked for medicinal use all year round: use a knife to cut the top of the root to harvest a rosette of leaves.

Plantain balm

A useful remedy for the relief of itching caused by insect bites, stings and nettle rash. Apply balm liberally to the affected area; if symptoms persist after a few hours, repeat application.

10 g (½ oz) beeswax

100 ml (3½ fl oz) plantain infused oil (see page 107)

5 drops lavender essential oil

You will also need: heatproof jug; pan; measuring jug; small, sterilized, lidded jars

1. Put the beeswax in a heatproof jug and place in a pan. Pour boiling water into the pan up to a level of about 5–10 cm (2–4 inch), taking care not to splash water on the wax. Turn on heat to a medium setting.

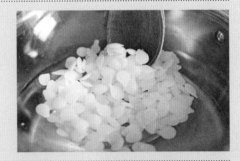

2. When the beeswax is dissolved, turn off the heat and pour in the plantain-infused oil. Stir gently to combine.

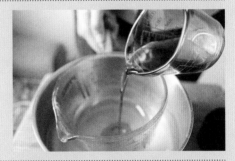

3. Add the lavender essential oil, stir gently, then, using oven gloves, pour immediately into small jars and seal. Use the balm within six months.

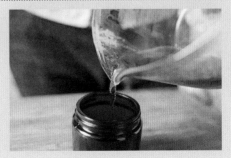

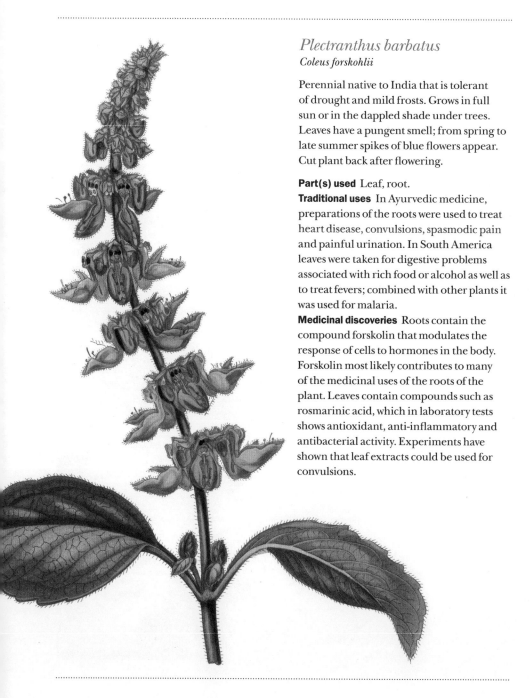

Plectranthus barbatus
Coleus forskohlii

Perennial native to India that is tolerant of drought and mild frosts. Grows in full sun or in the dappled shade under trees. Leaves have a pungent smell; from spring to late summer spikes of blue flowers appear. Cut plant back after flowering.

Part(s) used Leaf, root.

Traditional uses In Ayurvedic medicine, preparations of the roots were used to treat heart disease, convulsions, spasmodic pain and painful urination. In South America leaves were taken for digestive problems associated with rich food or alcohol as well as to treat fevers; combined with other plants it was used for malaria.

Medicinal discoveries Roots contain the compound forskolin that modulates the response of cells to hormones in the body. Forskolin most likely contributes to many of the medicinal uses of the roots of the plant. Leaves contain compounds such as rosmarinic acid, which in laboratory tests shows antioxidant, anti-inflammatory and antibacterial activity. Experiments have shown that leaf extracts could be used for convulsions.

Polygala senega
Senega

Perennial herb that is found across eastern N. America. Grow in a woodland or rock garden on wide range of soils in sun or semi-shade. The plant produces multiple stems each bearing a spike of green-white flowers in summer.

Part(s) used Root.
Traditional uses Used as an expectorant for treating coughs, acute bronchial catarrh and pneumonia. Also used to treat snake bites and rheumatism.
Medicinal discoveries Compounds called saponins in the roots could explain their use as an expectorant: they stimulate the bronchial mucous membranes, which triggers coughing and the removal of mucus.

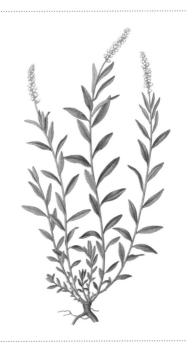

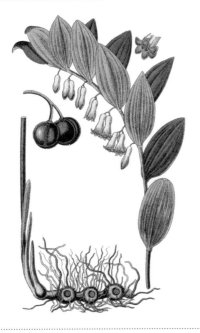

Polygonatum multiflorum
Solomon's seal

Hardy perennial with arching, leafy stems and cream flowers in late spring. Good plant for shade in moist but well-drained soil.

Part(s) used Rhizome.
Traditional uses King Solomon is said to have discovered the wound-healing properties of *Polygonatum* plants. The plant is a traditional Chinese medicine for heart problems, coughs and to promote secretion of body fluids. In Ayurvedic medicine, it was considered to be a rejuvenator and aphrodisiac. It was also reputed to aid fertility.
Medicinal discoveries Constituents of the rhizome have been investigated for effects on aiding the memory and prolonging life. Parts of the plant can be harmful if eaten.

Polygonum aviculare
Knotgrass, knotweed

Annual wasteland weed from temperate regions. Produces small pink-white flowers.

Part(s) used Aerial parts.
Traditional uses A folk remedy for respiratory-tract infections, catarrhs and coughs, with reputed expectorant effects. It was used to manage night sweats in those with tuberculosis. Also used as a diuretic, to treat skin problems and to control bleeding. It has been used in homeopathic remedies.
Medicinal discoveries Knotgrass has been investigated for its potential antiobesity effects and for its effects on blood pressure and cholesterol. Preparations have also been of interest to manage gum inflammation and infections.

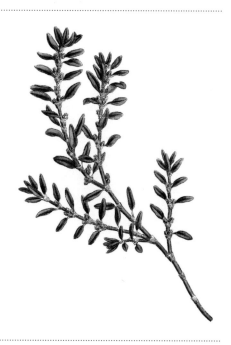

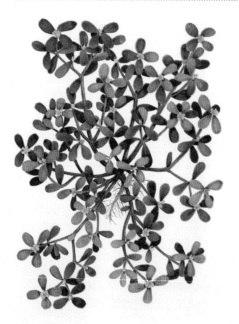

Portulaca oleracea
Purslane, pigweed

Annual with fleshy leaves and small yellow flowers. From regions in Asia but now distributed worldwide.

Part(s) used Aerial parts.
Traditional uses Known as a 'global panacea'. In traditional Chinese medicine it was given to cool the blood, reduce fevers and clear toxins. It was also a remedy for boils, eczema, stings and snake bites.
Medicinal discoveries A source of omega-3 fatty acids, which help maintain health. There has been interest for potential use in diabetes as studies suggest preparations may lower blood glucose. Preparations also have antibacterial properties and may help protect the liver and nerve cells.

Potentilla erecta
Tormentil

Perennial with small, bright yellow flowers occurring in regions of central and northern Europe, particularly in marshes, meadows and woods.

Part(s) used Rhizome.

Traditional uses Potentilla is derived from the Latin *potens*, meaning powerful, and refers to the plant's reputed medicinal effects. It was used as an astringent remedy for diarrhoea and as a gargle for mouth and throat inflammations. It was used for cholera and fevers, to alleviate haemorrhoids and aid the healing of wounds and ulcers. The herbalist Culpeper (see page 81) claimed of tormentil that it 'is most excellent to stay all fluxes of blood or humours, whether at nose, mouth or belly', and that it 'expels any venom or poison, or the plague', and that it also 'resisteth putrefaction'. These reputed actions might explain why the plant is also known as bloodroot.

Medicinal discoveries Scientific studies suggest preparations might help relieve diarrhoea. Preparations have antimicrobial properties and have been of interest to help prevent tooth decay. Other studies suggest preparations have antiviral, anti-inflammatory and anticancer properties. Tormentil has also been investigated in laboratory studies for its ability to reduce blood glucose. Therefore its potential antidiabetic effects are of interest.

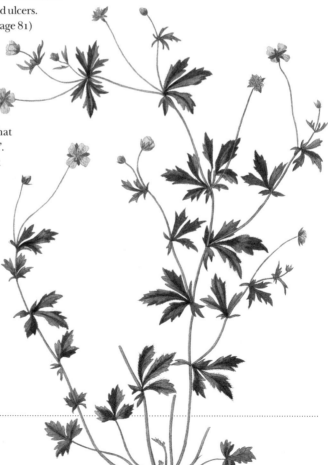

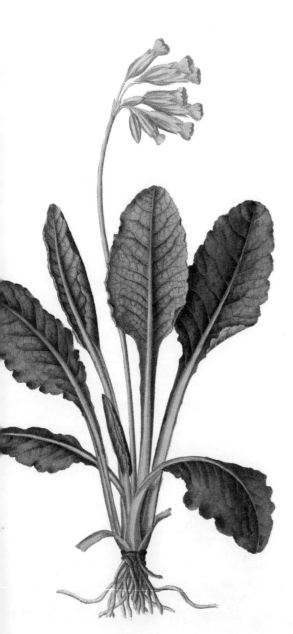

Primula veris
Cowslip

Hardy perennial native to temperate Europe and Asia. Usually one of the first flowers to bloom in spring, producing a cluster of fragrant, yellow flowers atop a slender stalk. Grows in open ground and in woods.

Part(s) used Flower, leaf, root.
Traditional uses Leaves were used to make a sedative tea to relieve the nerves and to help sleep. Roots were used as an expectorant to treat colds, flu-like symptoms and whooping cough. Aerial parts of the plant were also used to reduce blood clotting, as an analgesic, and in the treatment of rheumatic fevers, arthritis, tuberculosis, kidney complaints and urinary tract infections. Herbalists still make a lotion from cowslips for skin conditions including acne, pimples, and small wounds.
Medicinal discoveries Scientific studies have shown that cowslip has antispasmodic properties; further research is needed to evaluate whether the plant could be used to treat patients with epilepsy, tremors, and Parkinson's disease. Roots contain saponins that could explain its use as an expectorant.

Prunella vulgaris
Self-heal

Hardy perennial native to Europe, with creeping, self-rooting, reddish stems. Purple flowers appear in late spring until the autumn. Grows in grassy areas in most soils.

Part(s) used Aerial parts.
Traditional uses Traditionally made into a poultice for healing wounds. The herbalist Culpeper wrote that the plant is called self-heal because 'when you are hurt, you may heal yourself.' Herbalists use the plant for wounds and as a gargle for throat and mouth infections. In traditional Chinese medicine it is used for liver complaints.
Medicinal discoveries Scientific studies have shown that the plant has antiviral properties and has some mild anticancer activity.

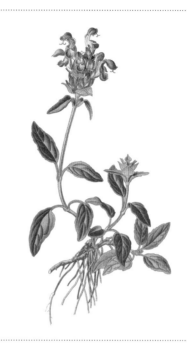

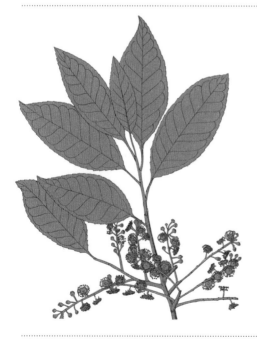

Prunus africana
Pygeum, African cherry

Tree indigenous to African rain forests. An endangered species, listed under the Convention on International Trade in Endangered Species of Wild Fauna and Flora.

Part(s) used Bark.
Traditional uses Used as a traditional African remedy for urinary, kidney and prostate problems, and to alleviate inflammation, malaria and fevers. It was also reputed to act as an aphrodisiac.
Medicinal discoveries Modern interest has focused on the potential for preparations to alleviate prostate disorders, particularly benign prostatic hyperplasia (enlarged prostate gland). Bark preparations also have anti-inflammatory properties.

Prunus spinosa
Blackthorn

Large deciduous shrub or small tree native to Europe and W. Asia. Flowers are creamy-white and produced shortly before the leaves in early spring. Autumn fruits (called sloes) are black with a purple-blue waxy shine.

Part(s) used Bark, flower, fruit.
Traditional uses Blackthorn was used as a diuretic, an astringent and antioxidant, to induce perspiration, reduce fever and treat stomach aches. Infusion from the flowers and fruit used as a tonic to purify the blood, prevent gout and relieve stomach aches and ease rheumatic pains.
Medicinal discoveries Scientific studies show that extracts have anti-inflammatory activity.

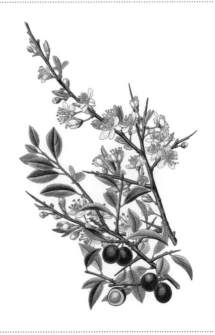

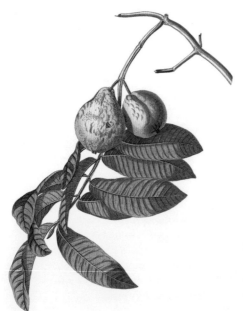

Psidium guajava
Guava

Tropical fruit tree from Central and S. America that produces white flowers and pear-shaped fruit. Important food crop.

Part(s) used Fruit, leaf.
Traditional uses Leaves were a traditional remedy for diabetes in Central America, South Africa and the Caribbean. In Central America they were also taken for skin disorders. In parts of Asia the plant was a remedy for digestive problems.
Medicinal discoveries Scientific studies show leaf preparations have anti-inflammatory and antimicrobial properties and that they may lower blood glucose. Flavonoid constituents have also shown effects on maintaining blood glucose levels.

Pueraria montana var. *lobata*
Kudzu vine

A deciduous vine from China and Japan. Its rapid growth rate and deep roots make it an invasive pest in parts of Europe and America. It can tolerate drought and shade, although the fragrant purple flowers may not appear in these conditions.

Part(s) used Root.

Traditional uses Dried kudzu vine root is a traditional Chinese medicine that has been used to treat fevers, headaches and dizziness and as a remedy for diarrhoea. It was used to quench thirst and to promote the eruption of measles spots, to alleviate heart pain and to remove 'wine toxin damaging the middle'. In traditional Korean medicine, the root was used to treat nerve disorders and the symptoms of Parkinson's disease.

Medicinal discoveries Scientific studies have revealed that the root of the kudzu vine contains compounds called isoflavones, which have oestrogen-like properties. There has been interest in the use of root preparations to relieve menopausal symptoms, to improve memory, particularly during the menopause, and to help preserve nerve cells in the brain.

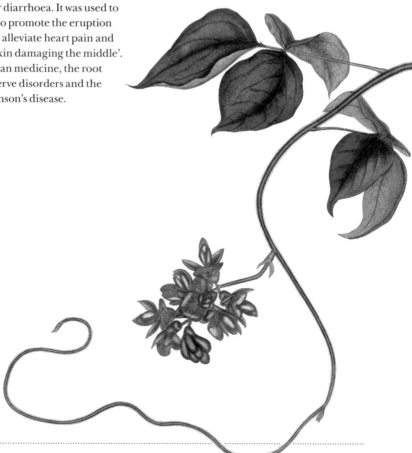

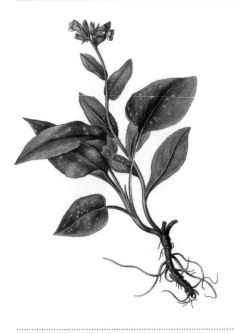

Pulmonaria officinalis
Lungwort

Evergreen perennial native to Europe. Spring–early summer flowers are red-pink turning blue-purple. Grows in shady areas.

Part(s) used Leaf.

Traditional uses According to the medieval Doctrine of Signatures (see page 81), the plant's spotted leaves were thought to represent diseased lungs and were used to treat chest diseases such as bronchitis and asthma. Used in herbal and homeopathic remedies to treat bronchitis, coughs and diarrhoea.

Medicinal discoveries Scientific studies have shown that leaves have a high mucilage content which can explain their traditional use in treating sore throats.

Pulsatilla vulgaris
Pasque flower, pulsatilla

Hardy, perennial, alpine plant, native to Europe. Bell-shaped, purple flowers appear before its leaves. Attractive seedheads.

Part(s) used Aerial parts.

Traditional uses Reputed to have relaxing properties, pasque flower was taken to aid sleep and ease nervous tension. It was also taken for earaches, headaches, respiratory infections, coughs, asthma, skin infections, such as boils, and menstrual pain.

Medicinal discoveries Pasque flower has been investigated for its effects on the womb. Components of this plant are suggested to have sedative and fever-reducing effects. The fresh plant is poisonous and contact with the plant may cause an allergic reaction.

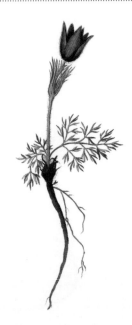

Quercus robur
Common oak

Slow-growing, deciduous tree native to
Europe. The long, drooping catkins are
male flowers; the short spikes are female
flowers (after pollination these develop
into the fruit, or acorn).

Part(s) used Bark.
Traditional uses All parts of the oak were
used to treat fevers, but the bark was used
for a wider range of conditions including
chronic diarrhoea, dysentery and nervous
disorders. It was also applied topically in
ointments to stop bleeding gums and piles.
Medicinal discoveries Bark shown to contain
a range of compounds with antibacterial
activity that could explain its traditional use
for stomach disorders.

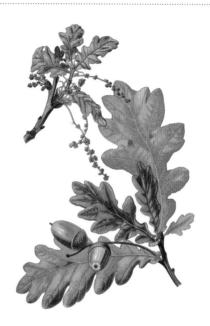

Rhamnus cathartica
Common buckthorn

Deciduous shrub or small tree native to
Europe and N. Africa. Glossy green leaves
turn yellow in autumn. Clusters of yellow
flowers in spring are followed by red berries
that ripen to black. Buckthorn's spine-tipped
shoots make it an ideal security hedge.

Part(s) used Fruit.
Traditional uses Used as a purgative in
the ninth century, especially for chronic
constipation. Also used to induce
perspiration and lower fever and to
treat gallstones, gout, rheumatism and
accumulation of fluid. Used topically to treat
skin diseases and the removal of warts.
Medicinal discoveries The fruit has been
found to have anti-inflammatory properties.

Rheum officinale
Chinese rhubarb

Perennial shrub native to China, thrives in full sun, in moist but not soggy soil. Leaves are triangular or heart-shaped and grow near the ground on reddish stalks. White or reddish-pink summer flowers.

Part(s) used Root, stalk.
Traditional uses Used as a laxative to relieve constipation and to treat stomach tumours. In traditional Chinese medicine it was prescribed for stomach disorders.
Medicinal discoveries The roots contain compounds with antibacterial and anti-yeast (*Candida*) activity. There is interest in the use of root and stalk material for use against hepatitis B.

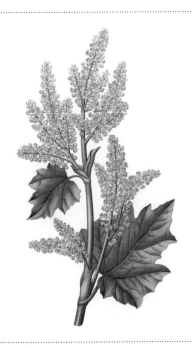

Ribes uva-crispa
Gooseberry

Deciduous shrub native to Europe, N.W. Africa and parts of Asia. In spring, it produces bell-shaped green flowers, which are followed by green fruits. There are cultivars with red, yellow or white fruits.

Part(s) used Fruit, leaf.
Traditional uses Fruits were used as a laxative and as a tonic to cleanse the system. Leaves were given for gravel and dysentery and as a poultice to heal wounds. Fresh fruits are still taken as a mild laxative.
Medicinal discoveries Scientific studies have shown the fruit and leaves contain compounds with antioxidant and antibacterial activity.

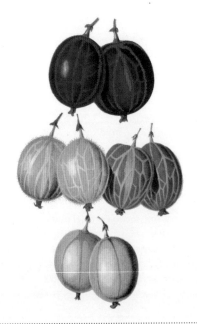

Weeds as medicine

The saying, 'A weed is simply a plant that is growing in the wrong place', reflects the social definition of a weed, which can vary depending on the value placed on a plant at a certain time. With the development of agriculture, with plants being bred to be bigger, sweeter and more showy, their wild ancestors are often dismissed as a nuisance – a weed to be removed, destroyed or ignored.

However, the use of plants as medicine began when all plants were wild, and many of the most popular plants used as remedies today are still found growing wild, such as stinging nettles (*Urtica* spp.), plantains (*Plantago* spp.), mints (*Mentha* spp.), dock leaves (*Rumex* spp.), and many more.

Most likely, the 'weedy' properties of these plants is what led them to be used so widely as medicines: weeds grow in disturbed ground, usually near areas of human activity; fast-growing and adaptable, they are readily available for much of the year. There is also a belief that wild plants are more effective than their cultivated counterparts; a belief that finds some scientific support in studies that show plants produce more of certain chemicals when under stress. Finally, weeds are plants that are well suited to their habitat, and so require little maintenance.

While it may be hard for some gardeners to start planting the very weeds they have been battling for so many years, rediscovering their medicinal value may make weeding much more interesting and, hopefully, productive.

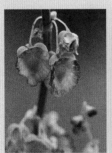
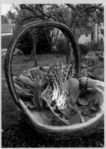

Left Seeds of french sorrel (*Rumex scutatus*).
Right Some common garden weeds picked to be used as medicine and food.

Rosa canina
Dog rose

The naval blockade during the Second World War meant that fruit imports weren't getting into the country. Concerned for the nation's health, Kew botanist Ronald Melville worked with the government to develop a rosehip syrup that would supply vital vitamin C. He found that the fruit (hips) of the dog rose are higher in vitamin C than other rose species. In 1941 a national collecting effort began and over 1,000 tons were gathered from the wild over the following four years. The practice of giving children rosehip syrup in winter continued into the 1960s.

During infections, the body quickly uses up its store of vitamin C and rosehips have long been considered beneficial for colds, flu and during convalescence. Vitamin C is essential for making collagen and is found in tendons and ligaments, which explains the traditional recommendation of rosehip syrup for rheumatic pain. The hips are also taken for diarrhoea and gastritis. Rosehip seed oil, which is high in essential fatty acids and antioxidants, is used for reducing the appearance of scars and stretch marks. In ninth century Italy, sniffing dried rose petals was said to fortify the brain and heart and restore the spirits.

Grow The dog rose requires full sun and something to climb on. It is adaptable to all soils and aspects. Flowers in early summer.
Harvest If using petals, remove those that have opened, leaving the centre to develop into fruit. Pick hips after the first frost or when some of them have started to soften.
Caution Seeds can aggravate the throat and skin.

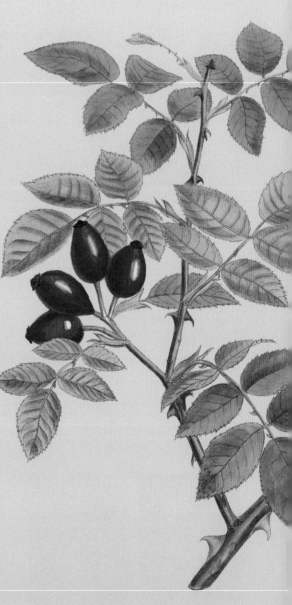

Rosehip syrup

For the best flavour and highest levels of vitamin C, it's best to use the hips of the dog rose, although the fruits from cultivated roses will do. Take a dessertspoonful of the syrup twice a day during the winter – either on its own, in a little warm water or added to a bowl of porridge.

150 g (5 oz) rosehips

500 ml (17 fl oz) water

Approximately 400 g (14 oz) sugar

You will also need: food processor; scales; saucepan; clean muslin; funnel; measuring jug; sterilized; bottle with stopper

1. Blitz the rosehips for a few seconds in a food processor.

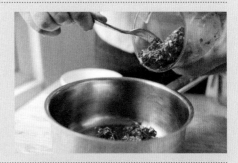

2. Spoon the rosehips into a saucepan, pour over the water and bring to the boil. Continue to boil for 10 minutes then cover the pan and leave for an hour. When cool, strain the liquid through a muslin-lined funnel into a measuring jug.

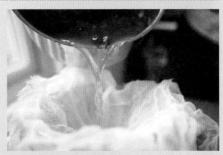

3. Take a note of the amount of liquid and pour it back into the cleaned saucepan. For every 30 ml (1 fl oz) of liquid add 30 g (1 oz) sugar. Dissolve the sugar over a gentle heat, simmer for five minutes, then turn off the heat and allow the syrup to cool. Pour the syrup into the bottle. Store in a cool dark place. It will keep for one year.

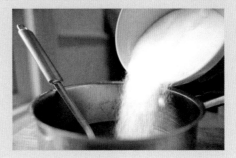

Rosmarinus officinalis
Rosemary

'There's rosemary, that's for remembrance;
pray, love, remember.' (*Hamlet* Act IV Sc V)
Ophelia's words are corroborated by
recent research at Northumbria University
which shows that smelling rosemary
essential oil can give a boost to mental
performance. It does this in a range of ways,
improving long-term memory, prospective
memory (remembering to complete a
task in the future) and mental arithmetic.
Taken internally it affects chemical
messages in the brain in a way that may
help with depression.

Surgeon to the Roman army Pedanius
Dioscorides in his text on medicines,
De Materia Medica, recommends rosemary
for jaundice, before exercise and for the
removal of fatigue. He also described it
as 'warming', and the seventeeth-century
herbalist Culpeper (see page 81) writes:
'[it helps] cold diseases of the head and
brain... drowsiness or dullness of the mind.'
Rosemary has a reputation for improving
circulation to the head and is used to treat
nervous tension, low mood and headache.
The effect on circulation is also given as
explanation for its external use to boost hair
growth and reduce neuralgic and sciatic
pain. It is also an ingredient in muscle rubs.
As with many aromatic herbs in the mint
family, rosemary is used for digestion and to
reduce gut spasms, as well as demonstrating
antibacterial and antioxidant action.

Grow Rosemary does best in sheltered, sunny
conditions in well-drained soil. It flowers
from early spring through to late autumn.
Harvest Cut only into new green growth.

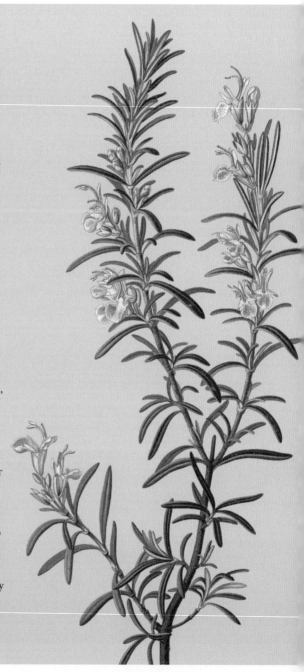

Rosemary-infused oil

*Apply the oil liberally as a muscle rub –
you may wish to add a few drops of your
favourite essential oils. Can be mixed with
beeswax to make a balm for the same purpose
(see page 43), or used as a hair oil.*

50 g (1¾ oz) dried rosemary sprigs

300 ml (10 fl oz) of olive oil

Vitamin E oil

**You will also need: pan; a heatproof bowl;
measuring jug; clean muslin; funnel; sterilized
bottle with stopper**

1. To prepare a water bath, choose a
heatproof bowl that will fit neatly into a
saucepan without its base coming into
contact with the pan. Working over the
bowl, strip the leaves from the sprigs,
then crumble the stems and leaves as finely
as you can. Pour over the oil.

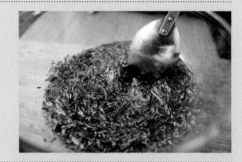

2. Add sufficient boiling water to the
saucepan so the bowl just sits in hot water.
Cover with a loose-fitting lid and heat very
gently for three hours, taking care not to
heat to bubbling point.

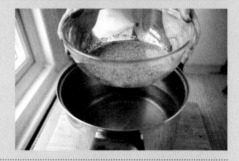

3. When cool, pour the mixture through a
muslin-lined funnel into a sterilized bottle.
Add three drops of vitamin E oil (to help
preserve it) and shake gently. Store in a cool,
dark place or in the fridge and use within
three months.

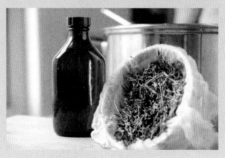

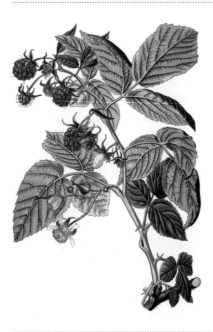

Rubus idaeus
Raspberry

Eurasian deciduous perennial shrub now widespread. Often with prickly stems. Cone-shaped, red to yellow, juicy fruit.

Part(s) used Leaf.
Traditional uses Leaves were reputed to strengthen the womb during pregnancy and labour. They were also considered to have astringent and antidiarrhoeal properties. Gargles and mouth washes were a remedy for ulcers, sore gums and throats, and a lotion was applied to alleviate conjunctivitis.
Medicinal discoveries Current interest has focused on the actions of leaf preparations on the womb, and their potential to alleviate menstrual symptoms. It is not recommended for use during pregnancy or labour.

Rumex crispus
Yellow dock

Perennial native to Europe and western Asia. Grows in a wide range of habitats from waste ground to shorelines. Green flowers on tall stalks bloom in the summer.

Part(s) used Leaves, root.
Traditional uses Root used to treat anaemia often used in combination with *Urtica dioica*. Leaves used as a poultice to counteract the stings from nettles as well as to treat skin sores and inflammation of the joints. Infusion of the roots was used to treat athlete's foot. Used in herbal remedies as a general tonic and in homeopathy for respiratory conditions.
Medicinal discoveries Extracts have anti-inflammatory properties.

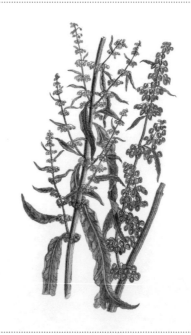

Ruscus aculeatus
Butcher's broom, box holly

Small, evergreen, perennial shrub with dark green, spiky foliage. Female plants produce red berries in late autumn to winter. Occurs across southern Europe, often in woodland.

Part(s) used Rhizome, root.

Traditional uses Preparations made from the rhizome and root were a traditional remedy for varicose veins, haemorrhoids, fluid retention and arthritis. Preparations were also applied as a compress to alleviate chilblains and to counteract warts. In addition, butcher's broom was considered to have laxative effects. The Ancient Greek physician Dioscorides described the plant as a remedy for kidney stones.

Medicinal discoveries Most scientific studies have focused on the potential for butcher's broom to help vein and circulation problems, including pain and heaviness in the legs, cramps in the calves, leg swelling and itching. Some studies suggest that root preparations might help alleviate these symptoms when taken as a herbal medicine and when applied to the legs as a cream. Ointment and suppository preparations are said to reduce symptoms of haemorrhoids. Root preparations have also been investigated for their potential to alleviate symptoms in premenstrual syndrome. Other studies have shown butcher's broom preparations to have anti-inflammatory, antibacterial and antifungal properties.

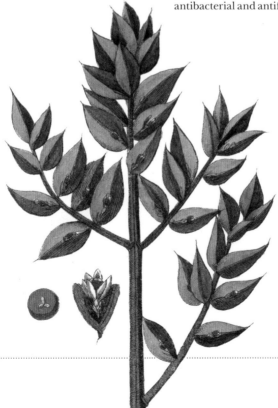

Salix alba
White willow

Fast-growing, deciduous tree native to Europe and western and central Asia. Underside of the leaves have a white appearance; the clusters of tiny flowers are called catkins. The tree grows in most soils but thrives near water. Cultivars differ in their physical form.

Part(s) used Bark, leaf.

Traditional uses Long history of use for the treatment of pain, to ease aches, reduce fevers, treat respiratory problems including catarrh and as an antiseptic. Extracts from willow are currently being used in cosmetics as well as many health products.

Medicinal discoveries In an early clinical trial, undertaken in 1763 by the Reverend Edward Stone from Oxfordshire, bark extracts were shown to reduce malarial fever. Many of the traditional uses of willow that involve the treatment of pain associated with inflammation can be explained by the presence of salicin. The body turns this compound into salicylic acid, which has pain-relieving properties. More recent clinical trials have shown that a bark extract was significantly better in treating pain in patients with osteoarthritis than a placebo.

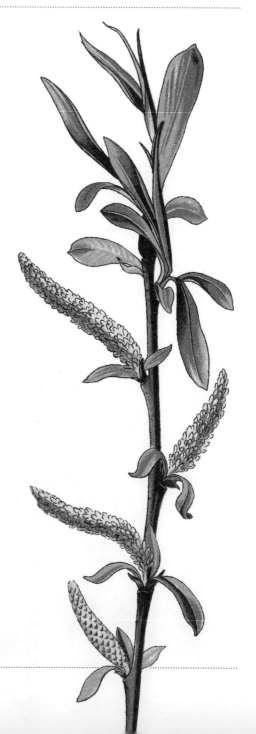

Salvia officinalis
Sage

Aromatic, evergreen perennial with grey-green leaves and blue-mauve flowers in early summer. Sage makes a decorative garden shrub that will tolerate cool climates.

Part(s) used Leaf.

Traditional uses Sage has a longstanding reputation in traditional European herbal medicine for its antiseptic and anti-inflammatory properties and has been used as a remedy for sore throats and inflammation of the mouth and gums. It was reputed to reduce sweating and to alleviate digestive complaints such as flatulence. The sixteenth-century herbalist John Gerard (see page 81) claimed sage was 'singularly good for the head and brain and quickenethe the nerves and memory'.

Medicinal discoveries There has been much interest in the potential for sage to aid the memory. Several scientific studies show that preparations of the common garden sage (*S. officinalis*) and the Spanish sage (*S. officinalis* subsp. *lavandulifolia*) can improve learning and memory. Both types of sage could also improve the symptoms of Alzheimer's disease. Sage preparations have anti-inflammatory and antioxidant effects, and might also improve nerve function and protect nerve cells. Sage has also been investigated for its ability to reduce sweating, particularly during the menopause.

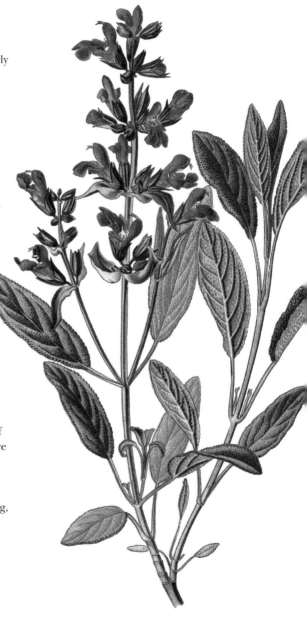

Sambucus nigra
Elder

The elder tree has something of a split personality: both shrouded in superstition (it was thought to bring bad luck if brought indoors) and respected for its many healing properties. It is a fast-growing tree with a distinctive spongy centre that is easily removed, lending the branches to use as a wind instrument in ancient times.

The flowers are traditionally used to treat hayfever, often in combination with nettle, yarrow, eyebright and peppermint. The remedy is considered most effective if taken regularly as a strong tea a month before the hayfever season begins. The main use of the berry is as a cold and flu cure. Recent research suggests that elderberry can stop viruses from attaching to your airways and thus prevent them from becoming established. It is often taken in the form of a syrup, which has the added benefit of soothing an itchy infected throat.

Grow Grows in sun or semi-shade in hedgerows and woodland edges. Prefers a nitrogen-rich, moisture-retentive soil. Cut back up to 1 m (3¼ ft) of growth every two to three years.
Harvest Pick flowers on a sunny day when they are covered in yellow pollen and smell fresh. Use newly harvested flowers to make cordials, or dry them to make teas and tinctures. Pick berries when they are dark purple and soft. They can be frozen.
Caution Leaves and branches are poisonous.

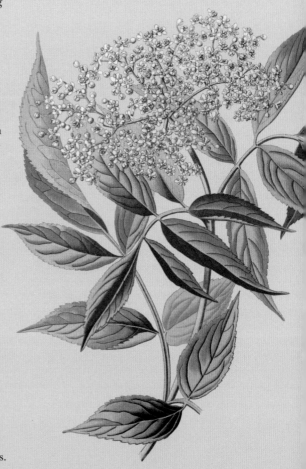

Elderberry vinegar

A great way to enjoy both the flavour and medicinal actions of elderberries is to make an infused vinegar. Whisk it into salad dressings, use it as a marinade for meat or add it to gravy and sauces. At the first sign of a cold or flu, take one teaspoonful three times a day.

300 g (10½ oz) elderberries

250 ml (9 fl oz) cider or white wine vinegar

30 g (1 oz) muscovado sugar

You will also need: scales; fork; saucepan; measuring jug; potato masher; clean muslin; funnel; sterilized bottle with stopper

1. Use the tines of a fork to remove the berries from their stalks (this is less messy if you freeze them first). Do this directly over a bowl to catch any juice.

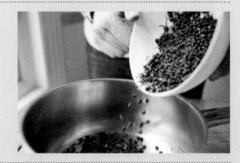

2. Pour over the vinegar and heat the mixture on a low heat with the lid on for 30 minutes then leave for two hours.

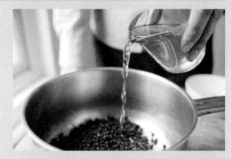

3. Pulp the berries using a potato masher. Return the saucepan to the heat, add the sugar and continue stirring until dissolved. Allow to cool slightly before pouring the mixture through a muslin-lined funnel into sterilized bottles. Will keep for two years.

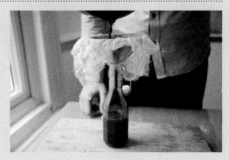

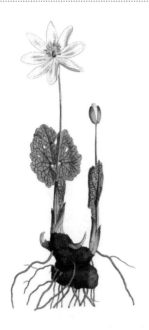

Sanguinaria canadensis
Bloodroot

Perennial found in woodlands in N. America. Cup-shaped, white flowers open before the leaves in early spring. Cultivars are available with double flowers. Does best in reliably moist soil in site with sun only part of the day.

Part(s) used Rhizome.
Traditional uses Long historical use as an emetic and to treat respiratory conditions.
Medicinal discoveries Scientific studies have shown that bloodroot contains sanguinarine, a benzylisoquinoline alkaloid, which has antibacterial properties. Products containing sanguinarine have been used in toothpastes as an antibacterial to prevent plaque formation.

Sanguisorba officinalis
Great burnet

Hardy herbaceous perennial from temperate areas in the northern hemisphere. Attractive green foliage turns red in autumn. Small rounded maroon flower spikes are produced in summer and early autumn. Prefers moist but well-drained soil in sun or partial shade.

Part(s) used Aerial parts.
Traditional uses Culpepper (see page 81) wrote that the stalks 'quicken the spirits, refresh and cheer the heart, and drive away melancholy'. It is used in traditional Chinese medicine to cool the blood, stop bleeding, clear heat and heal wounds.
Medicinal discoveries Compounds in the leaves and flowers have shown anti-inflammatory properties.

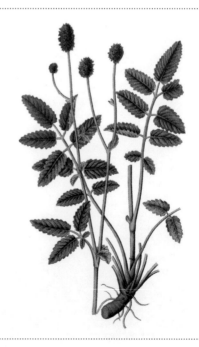

Sanicula europaea
Wood sanicle

European perennial with dark green, lobed leaves and white-pinkish summer flowers. Grows in shady places.

Part(s) used Root.
Traditional uses As a treatment for disorders of the gastrointestinal and respiratory tracts, also taken for mild lung inflammation and congestion, coughs and bronchitis. Used topically for skin problems, haemorrhoids and to stop nose bleeds. Tea made from the roots taken as a carminative tonic, an expectorant and as a gargle for sore throats.
Medicinal discoveries Contains saponins and phenolic compounds that could explain some of its medicinal properties.

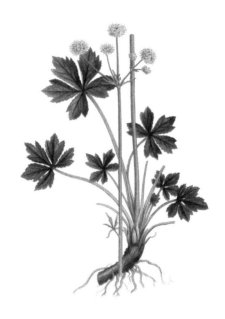

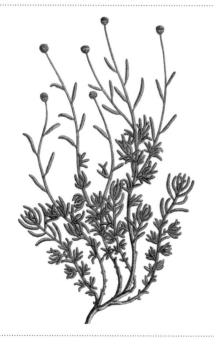

Santolina chamaecyparissus
Cotton lavender

Dwarf evergreen, Mediterranean shrub with aromatic silver-grey leaves and yellow flowers.

Part(s) used Aerial parts.
Traditional uses Culpeper (see page 81) wrote that cotton lavender 'resists poison, putrefaction and heals the biting of venomous beasts'. The juice was used to bathe the eyes, the plant to treat worms in children and the twigs to repel moths.
Medicinal discoveries Cotton lavender is suggested to have anti-inflammatory and anti-ulcer properties and might modulate the function of the immune system. These effects have not been confirmed in studies in humans. The oil has been investigated for antimicrobial effects.

Satureja hortensis
Summer savory

Annual, native to N. Africa, southern parts of
Europe, Middle East and Central Asia. Has
tubular, lilac flowers in summer with bronze-
green leaves. Grow as an edging plant.

Part(s) used Aerial parts.
Traditional uses Used medicinally to treat
digestive problems, muscle and bone
pain and different infectious diseases. It
was thought savory made people thin and
prevented flatulence. English colonists
took it with them to N. America as a cure for
diarrhoea (it was made into a tea).
Medicinal discoveries Essential oil from
the leaves contains thymol which has anti-
inflammatory and antimicrobial activity.

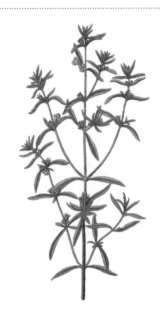

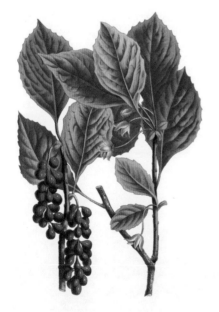

Schisandra chinensis
Magnolia vine

Deciduous climber that grows wild in
China, Japan and Korea. Produces fragrant
cream or pale pink flowers from late spring
followed by pink or red fruit.

Part(s) used Fruit.
Traditional uses A traditional Chinese
medicine given for breathing difficulties and
coughs, and to reduce sweating and frequent
urination. Fruits were also used to alleviate
diarrhoea, palpitations and insomnia.
They were also considered a stimulating
and fortifying tonic for physical exhaustion.
Medicinal discoveries The fruits may help
protect the liver, counteract fatigue and
increase endurance. Also of interest are
potential anticancer and antioxidant effects.

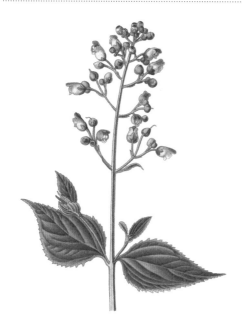

Scrophularia nodosa
Knotted figwort

Perennial found in northern temperate areas in Europe and Asia. Grows in moist woodland, near streams and in hedgerows. Leaves have an unpleasant aroma, summer flowers are green-brown.

Part(s) used Leaf.
Traditional uses According to the Doctrine of Signatures (see page 81), the plant was thought to be able to cure the throat disease scrofula because of the throat-like shape of its flowers. It was also made into a poultice to treat wounds and taken as a tonic to boost poor circulation.
Medicinal discoveries Leaves contain compounds called iridoid glycosides that have wound-healing properties.

Scutellaria baicalensis
Helmet flower, skullcap

Bushy perennial from E. Asia with purple flowers. *S. lateriflora* is a perennial indigenous to N. America.

Part(s) used Root.
Traditional uses *S. baicalensis* root is a traditional Chinese medicine taken for nausea, vomiting and diarrhoea, also for coughs, fevers, allergies, sores and swellings. *S. lateriflora* was considered a mild sedative, reputed to treat rabies, and taken for nervous conditions and seizures.
Medicinal discoveries The root has anti-inflammatory and anti-allergic properties. There is interest in its potential for lowering cholesterol. *S. lateriflora* is of interest to improve mood and reduce anxiety.

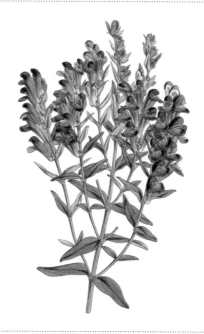

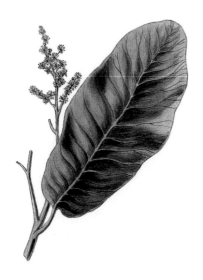

Semecarpus anacardium
Oriental cashew

Deciduous tree found in central India and the sub-Himalayan region.

Part(s) used Fruit, seed.

Traditional uses Fruits were a traditional Indian medicine, taken as a tonic and aphrodisiac. They were said to control flatulence, worms and asthma, aid nervous disorders and help arthritis.

Medicinal discoveries Modern interest has focused on the seeds' anti-inflammatory properties; preparations have been investigated for their benefits for arthritis and are suggested to have antifungal and antioxidant properties. The seed oil has been investigated for anticancer effects.

Sempervivum tectorum
Houseleek

Evergreen, succulent perennial with fleshy leaves and mauve-red flowers. Occurs in mountainous regions of Europe and is naturalized in the UK.

Part(s) used Leaf.

Traditional uses Leaves were applied as a poultice to burns, contusions, ulcers and inflamed skin. Juice was applied as a remedy for warts and corns. Culpeper (see page 81) claimed houseleek 'easeth the headache, and the distempered heat of the brain in frenzies, or want of sleep'. Houseleeks were planted on roofs to protect from lightning.

Medicinal discoveries Scientific studies suggest houseleeks might have pain-relieving and anti-inflammatory properties.

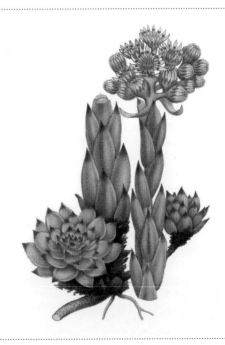

Senna alexandrina
Alexandrian senna

Frost-tender, deciduous shrub, native to
N. Africa and Asia. Grows in full sun on
sandy soils. Produces yellow pea-like flowers
in the summer followed by pods.

Part(s) used Leaf, pod.
Traditional uses Leaves and pods have a
long historical use as a laxative.
Medicinal discoveries The active
ingredients in senna pods and leaves are
the sennosides. They are broken down by
the bacteria in the colon to compounds
which stimulate peristalsis (wave-like
contractions of the colon) and emptying
of the colon. Many senna pod-based
products are available as laxatives.

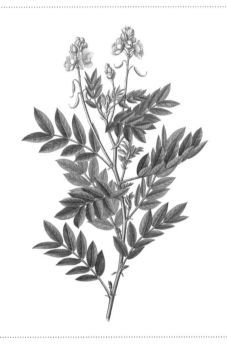

Serenoa repens
Saw palmetto

Shrub-like palm, indigenous to Florida,
with fan-shaped leaves and fragrant white
spring flowers.

Part(s) used Fruit.
Traditional uses Fruits were a remedy for
urine infections, such as cystitis, and were
reputed to have diuretic properties. They
were also used to tone and strengthen the
male reproductive system and were taken as
a sedative and tonic for the nervous system.
Medicinal discoveries Current interest in
the fruit is focused on treating symptoms of
enlarged prostate glands, specifically benign
prostatic hyperplasia. Studies suggest that
the fruits have anti-inflammatory effects and
may counteract fluid retention.

Seriphidium cinum
Wormseed

Deciduous, perennial aromatic shrub native to China. Grows in dry sandy desert type soils, can be grown in a rockery in full sun.

Part(s) used Flower.

Traditional uses In traditional Chinese and Ayurvedic medicines, wormseed was given as a mild anthelmintic (drug that expels parasites from the body) and digestive. It was also used to treat fevers, as an aid to digestion and for nervous disorders.

Medicinal discoveries The compound called santonin was isolated from the plant and used as an anthelmintic. However, it is no longer used as there are safer alternatives.

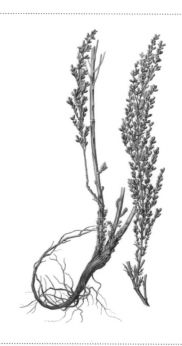

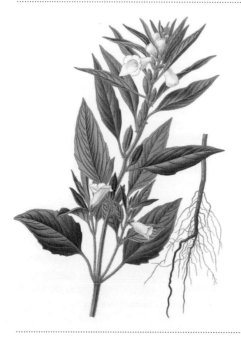

Sesamum indicum
Sesame

Frost-tender annual from Africa and India with tubular flowers that vary in colour from white to purple. Needs full sun; prefers a moist soil. Widely grown for its edible seeds.

Part(s) used Leaf, seed, seed oil.

Traditional uses Used to treat cardiovascular, gastrointestinal and respiratory ailments. Seeds and fresh leaves were made into a poultice to treat skin conditions.

Medicinal discoveries Seeds contain the compounds sesamin and sesamolin that can in experimental conditions lower cholesterol levels and high blood pressure. Oil has antimicrobial activity and has been added to ointments for athlete's foot.

Silybum marianum
Milk thistle, lady's thistle

Biennial found in Mediterranean regions, and parts of Europe, Africa and Asia; naturalized in the Americas and Australia.Often grown for its attractive, heavily veined leaves and purple, thistle-like flowers.

Part(s) used Fruit, leaf.
Traditional uses Fruits and leaves have been taken traditionally for liver and gall bladder disorders, including jaundice. Fruits were thought to aid milk production and treat haemorrhoids and stomach complaints, such as bloating and flatulence. A soothing remedy was made from the fruits for coughs and catarrh. In traditional Chinese medicine, fruits have been used for liver disorders and for hypochondriac pain. Leaves were taken for menstrual complaints and as an antimalarial remedy.
Medicinal discoveries There has been much interest, especially in Germany, in the use of the fruits as a remedy for liver disorders. Some scientific studies suggest they may protect the liver and aid liver regeneration. Other research suggests that some flavonoid components in the fruit have anticancer properties, and they might help protect against gastric ulcers and improve elasticity of the skin. Fruits have also shown antioxidant and anti-inflammatory properties.

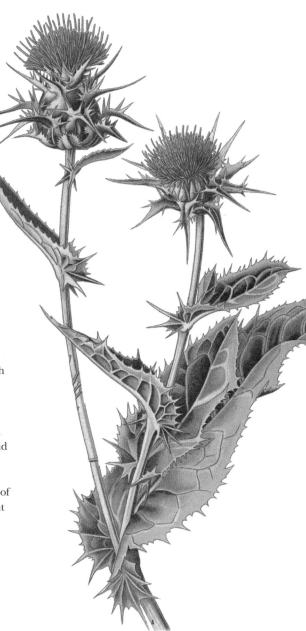

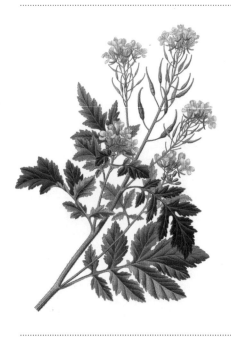

Sinapis alba
White mustard

Mediterranean annual naturalized in Britain. Produces small yellow flowers in midsummer followed by seeds.

Part(s) used Seed.
Traditional uses Recommended by Culpeper (see page 81) for weak stomachs, toothache, joint pains and cricks in the neck. For muscle aches, plaster preparations were applied to the skin. In traditional Chinese medicine, seeds were a remedy for coughs and colds, chest pains, joint numbness and abscesses.
Medicinal discoveries Seed preparations are applied to joints for rheumatic disorders and have been investigated for use in psoriasis, asthma and bronchitis. May cause an allergic reaction when applied to the skin.

Sinomenium acutum
Orient vine

A deciduous climber native to China and other regions in Asia.

Part(s) used Stem.
Traditional uses The stem has been used in traditional Chinese medicine as a remedy for fevers, allergies, numbness, itching and joint swellings associated with arthritis.
Medicinal discoveries Scientific studies have shown that stem preparations have anti-inflammatory properties, which might explain their traditional use for arthritis. Other studies suggest that chemical components of the stems might have anti-allergic and anticancer effects

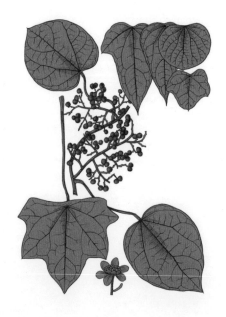

Sisymbrium officinale
Hedge mustard

An annual herbaceous plant, native to Britain, with a mustard-like fragrance.

Part(s) used Aerial parts.
Traditional uses A traditional remedy, popular with teachers and singers, to restore loss of voice. It was also used to alleviate breathing problems and treat urinary and gastrointestinal disorders. The Ancient Greeks and Romans thought it could combat growths associated with cancer.
Medicinal discoveries In some scientific studies, the plant has shown antibacterial, anti-inflammatory and antifungal properties. It has been investigated for its potential to help protect against cancer and to help relax the airways and aid breathing.

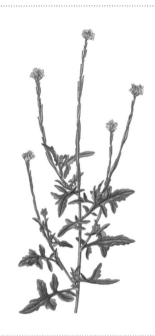

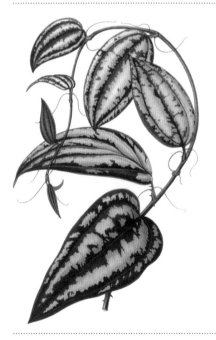

Smilax ornata
Sarsaparilla

An evergreen climber with small white-green flowers, followed by black berries. Different varieties and botanical sources of sarsaparilla are cultivated in regions of Central America as a flavouring for drinks.

Part(s) used Rhizome, root.
Traditional uses Sarsaparilla (*S. purhampuy* and *S. ornata*) was a reputed cure-all said to restore body functions and alleviate skin conditions such as psoriasis. It was also used as a remedy for itching, inflamed joints, syphilis and leprosy.
Medicinal discoveries Suggested to improve digestion and appetite and have some diuretic properties. It may have anti-inflammatory effects and help protect the liver.

Smyrnium olusatrum
Wild celery, Alexanders, horse parsley

Biennial native to Europe, although now
more widely distributed. Wayside plant with
lime green foliage and small yellow flowers
in summer.

Part(s) used Aerial parts, root.
Traditional uses Reputed to have diuretic
properties and to aid the digestive system.
Ancient Romans used it for both medicinal
and culinary purposes.
Medicinal discoveries The essential oil from
the aerial parts has shown antibacterial and
antifungal properties. The oil has been tested
for anticancer activity and plant constituents
have been investigated for their potential to
help protect the liver and nerve cells.

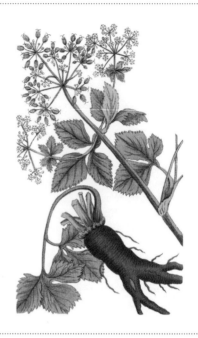

Solanum americanum
American black nightshade

Short-lived perennial that is distributed
throughout many parts of the world.
Grows on disturbed ground and wasteland.

Part(s) used Aerial parts.
Traditional uses Leaf preparations were
applied to the skin to relieve pain and
inflammation, and for burns and ulcers.
The juice was applied to treat ringworm, gout
and earache. In Bohemia, leaves were placed
in the cradles of infants to aid sleep. Also
long known for its poisonous properties.
Medicinal discoveries Although the herb has
been used in some liniments, poultices, and
decoctions for external application to ease
pain, it is rarely used for these medicinal
purposes now. Known to have toxic effects.

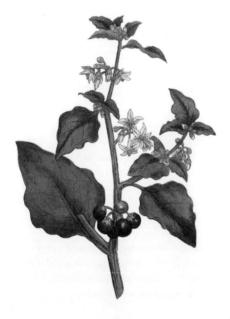

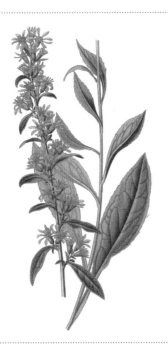

Solidago virgaurea
Goldenrod

Hardy perennial native to Europe. Plumes of yellow flowers are carried on tall stems in late summer. Makes a good back of the border plant.

Part(s) used Aerial parts.
Traditional uses Used to heal wounds, as a diuretic, and to treat tuberculosis, diabetes, enlarged liver, gout, haemorrhoids, internal bleeding, asthma, and arthritis. It was used as a rinse to treat mouth and throat inflammations. Taken as an infusion to treat urinary tract disorders.
Medicinal discoveries Extracts have anti-inflammatory and antibacterial activity that could explain some of its traditional uses.

Stachys officinalis
Wood betony

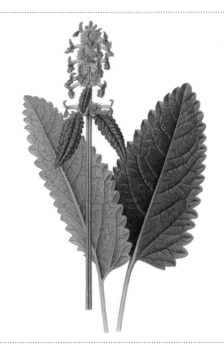

An upright perennial that occurs across parts of Europe, often in grassland and meadows. Produces red-purple flower spikes in summer and early autumn.

Part(s) used Flower, leaf.
Traditional uses Leaves and flowers were reputed to strengthen the nervous system and to relieve anxiety and tension. They were a remedy for insomnia, nightmares, headaches and neuralgia. Roots were used as a purgative and to induce vomiting.
Medicinal discoveries Leaf preparations have shown anti-inflammatory and antioxidant effects. The essential oil has antimicrobial properties and there has been interest in its use to treat fungal infections.

Stellaria media
Chickweed

Twelfth-century abbess and mystic Hildegard von Bingen recommended a warm chickweed poultice: 'If a person has fallen by accident, or has been struck by cudgels, so that his skin is bruised. . . It will dispel the mucus collected there'. Historically, chickweed is repeatedly referred to as 'soothing' and 'cooling'. Nowadays it is used as a traditional remedy for inflammations that feel hot or itchy, including sunburn, eczema, psoriasis and nettle rash. As a home remedy, freshly picked chickweed is applied directly, or pounded with a pestle and mortar, then held in place with a bandage or cling film.

Herbalist Richard Hool wrote in 1918, 'It is good in all cases of weakness, inflammation of the stomach and bowels, bronchial tubes, lungs, and for peritonitis, or any form of internal inflammation.' Chickweed is also reputed to reduce obesity when dried and taken as a tea. In the nineteenth century, chickweed juice was recommended for convalescence and to prevent scurvy. There is very little scientific research on the medicinal effects of this common weed, though it would have been effective against scurvy if enough was taken as, like most edible greens, it is rich in vitamin C. The fresh leaves are mild in flavour and balance the stronger tasting leaves in salad.

Grow Grows in bare, fertile, well-watered soil. Can be sown easily, though often appears of its own accord. Survives into winter but is frost-tender.
Harvest Pick any time as long as the leaves appear healthy.

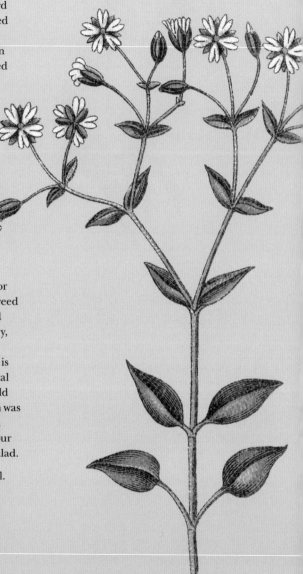

Chickweed cream

Use this cream to soothe inflamed, itchy skin.
Apply once or twice a day to the affected area.

Large bunch of fresh chickweed stems and leaves

Base cream

Peppermint (*Mentha* x *piperita*) essential oil

You will also need: juicer or blender; measuring jug;
clean muslin; small sterilized, lidded jars

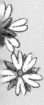

1. If you have a juicer, process the chickweed and collect the juice in a measuring jug. Alternatively, blitz the chickweed in a blender, spoon the pulp into the centre of the muslin square, wrap up tightly and squeeze, catching the juice in the jug. Discard the pulp.

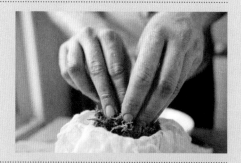

2. For every 10 ml (2 teaspoons) of juice you will need 30 g (1 oz) base cream. Mix together in a small bowl. If the mixture becomes too liquid add a little more cream. For every 100 g (3½ oz) of cream you use add 20 drops of peppermint essential oil.

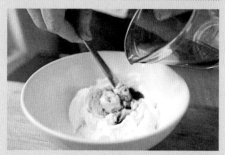

3. Spoon the cream into small sterilized jars. Store in the fridge for 3–6 months.

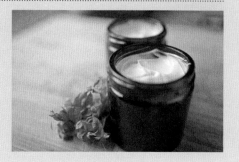

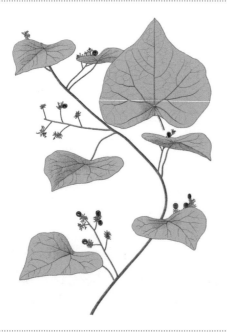

Stephania tetrandra
Han Fang Ji

Perennial twining vine native to China. Grows best in cool areas such as the edge of a wood. Small green flowers in late spring.

Part(s) used Root.

Traditional uses Used in traditional Chinese medicine to dispel wind and dampness, to relieve pain and promote diuresis (excretion of urine).

Medicinal discoveries Roots contain alkaloids such as tetrandrine that have been shown to increase urine production as well as being immunosuppressive, anti-inflammatory and antibacterial. Tetrandrine also expands coronary blood vessels, increasing blood flow and lowering blood pressure.

Sterculia urens
Gum karaya

Medium-sized deciduous tree native to India, found growing on dry, rocky hills. Has smooth, greenish-grey bark (which peels away in long, papery flakes), large lobed leaves and sprays of yellow-green flowers. Fruits have stinging hairs.

Part(s) used Resin.

Traditional uses Used as a laxative and reputed to have aphrodisiac properties.

Medicinal discoveries When the gum absorbs water it swells in volume. Studies have shown that if ingested, the gum adds bulk to the intestines, which helps explain its action as a laxative. The gum also has adhesive properties and is used for fixing dentures.

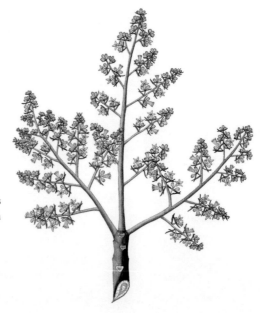

Styphnolobium japonicum
Japanese pagoda tree

Deciduous tree native to China. A popular street tree, it has bright green, fern-like leaves, and fragrant, white pea-like flowers in summer, followed by attractive pods. Needs full sun.

Part(s) used Flower, seed.
Traditional uses Long historical use as one of the fifty key plants used in traditional Chinese medicine for its antibacterial, anti-inflammatory, diuretic, emetic, emollient, febrifuge and purgative properties
Medicinal discoveries Laboratory-based studies have supported many of the traditional uses of the tree, but as yet there are few clinical studies on standardized extracts from the flowers and seeds.

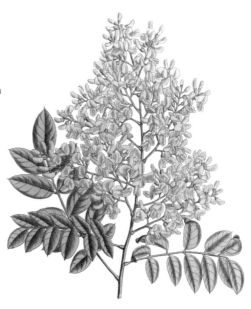

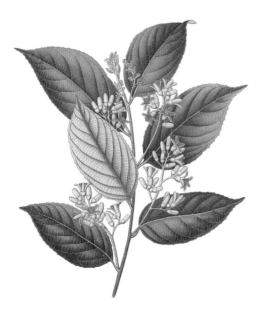

Styrax benzoin
Gum benzoin

Evergreen tree native to Indonesia. Bark is grey-brown and leaves are covered with a whitish down. Fragrant, silky white flowers in summer.

Part(s) used Bark, resin.
Traditional uses Used as a tincture to treat respiratory ailments, including asthma, bronchitis and throat infections. A mouthwash was taken for *Candida* infections. Used in dentistry as an anti-inflammatory after tooth extraction.
Medicinal discoveries Laboratory studies have shown the resin has antiseptic and anti-inflammatory properties, which can explain many of its traditional uses. The resin is used in cough and cold remedies.

Symphytum officinale
Comfrey

The word comfrey comes from the Latin *confervere*, to grow together. Its many common names, including woundwort, bruisewort and knitbone, record the plant's renown for healing wounds, sprains and broken bones. Comfrey has been well studied in trials, several of which support its efficacy in reducing back pain, inflammation caused by sprains, and for pain relief and increasing mobility in osteoarthritis of the knee.

It is thought to work by reducing inflammation and encouraging the growth of new connective tissue. Although inflammation is part of the healing process it can become chronic after injury causing swelling, pain and heat. A poultice made from boiled comfrey leaves is recorded, as recently as the mid-twentieth century, as a common treatment for swollen knees in Yorkshire mining communities. Herbalists advise against applying comfrey to a deep wound as it would heal over too rapidly. Comfrey contains toxic chemicals called pyrrolizidine alkaloids that can cause severe liver damage if taken internally. The level of alkaloids is ten times higher in the roots than the leaves. Traditionally leaves were ingested to heal ulcers and bleeding in the digestive and urinary tracts. However, comfrey is now only recommended for external use.

Grow Prefers damp, shady spots. Can spread quickly. Flowers in late spring to summer.
Harvest Leaves can be picked any time so long as they are looking healthy. Wear gloves.
Caution Don't use on broken skin. Do not take internally.

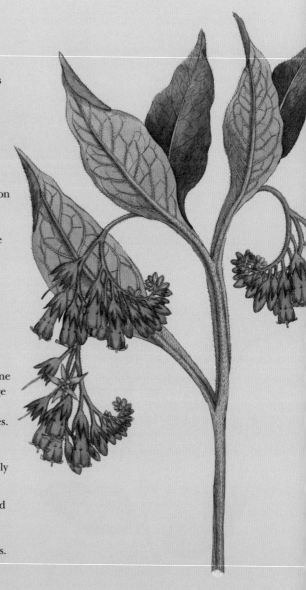

Comfrey ointment

Comfrey ointment is traditionally used for bruises, sprains and on joints affected by osteoarthritis. The frankincense augments the anti-inflammatory effect and acts as a preservative. Apply the ointment liberally twice a day to the affected area. Can also be used for rough hands.

10 g (½ oz) beeswax

20 g (¾ oz) coconut oil

90 ml (3 fl oz) comfrey infused oil (see page 107)

Thirty drops frankincense (*Boswellia sacra*) oil

You will also need: scales; heatproof bowl; saucepan; oven gloves; small sterilized jars with lids

1. Put the beeswax and coconut oil in a heatproof bowl. Stand the bowl in a large saucepan of boiling water over a gentle heat. Stir the mixture occasionally until it has melted together to form a liquid then stir in the comfrey infused oil.

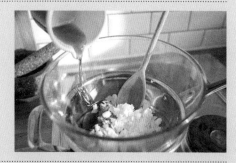

2. Wearing oven gloves, remove the bowl from the heat and stir in the essential oil. Allow to cool slightly.

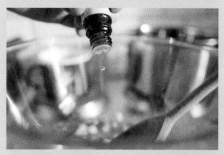

3. While it is still liquid, pour the mixture into sterilized jars. Store for up to one year.

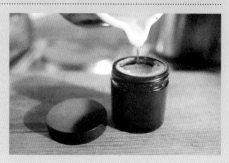

Syringa vulgaris
Lilac

Hardy, deciduous shrub from E. Europe with many horticultural cultivars. Lilacs do well in most soils, but will thrive on chalk, in full sun or light shade. The fragrant, spring blossom is widely used as a cut flower.

Part(s) used Essential oil from flower.
Traditional uses Used as a tonic to treat fevers and to rid the intestines of parasitic worms. The essential oil was used to treat skin ailments such as rashes, sunburns and minor cuts.
Medicinal discoveries Scientific studies have shown the oil contains compounds that have a calming effect that could help ease anxiety.

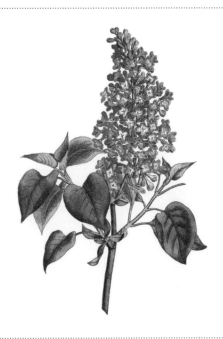

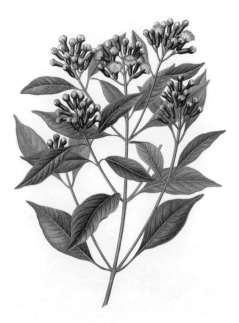

Syzygium aromaticum
Cloves

A tree with aromatic flowers, native to the Indonesian Moluccas Islands. Now grown widely as a commercial crop in the tropics.

Part(s) used Flower bud.
Traditional uses Prepared as a tonic to relieve sickness and flatulence. The oil was used as a remedy for toothache. In traditional Chinese medicine, cloves have been used for hiccups, diarrhoea and stomach pains.
Medicinal discoveries Clove oil has mild anaesthetic and antiseptic properties. It is used in dentistry to relieve toothache. There is interest in its use to prevent tooth plaque. Clove oil may have antihistamine, antispasmodic and antiviral effects. It can also be an irritant when applied.

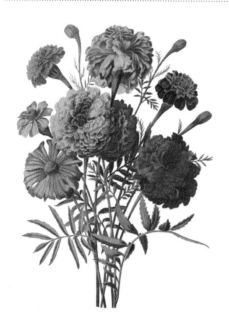

Tagetes erecta
African marigold, American marigold

Ornamental annual that occurs as various cultivars with yellow, orange and bronze flowers. It needs sun and prefers well-drained soils.

Part(s) used Flower.
Traditional uses Flowers were reputed to treat skin problems, including sores, wounds, burns, ulcers, boils and eczema. Flower preparations were given for piles, constipation, kidney disorders, muscle aches and earache. Petals have been eaten in salads.
Medicinal discoveries In studies, flower preparations have shown pain-relieving and antioxidant effects. There is interest in them for skin ailments and for use in cosmetics, as they may help protect skin.

Tamus communis
Black bryony

A perennial climber that grows in woodlands and hedgerows in Britain and parts of Europe. Prefers moist soil.

Part(s) used Fruit, root.
Traditional uses Roots and berries were used in folk medicine in Algeria for conditions associated with pain and inflammation, including rheumatism and lumbago. They were also said to counteract skin problems.
Medicinal discoveries Studies suggest root preparations have anti-inflammatory and pain-relieving properties, so have been investigated for their ability to alleviate gout. Root constituents have shown antiviral effects. The plant and fruits can cause irritation and dermatitis on contact.

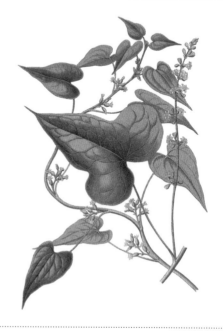

Tanacetum parthenium
Feverfew

Aromatic perennial herb with daisy-like flowers and ferny foliage. Considered native to S.E. Europe and W. Asia. Widely occurs throughout Europe and N. and S. America.

Part(s) used Leaf.

Traditional uses Feverfew was taken for fevers and pain, particularly for arthritis and migraines, but also for stomach aches and toothaches. The plant was used for menstrual disorders, menopausal symptoms and during labour. Was thought to aid digestion, boost appetite, and cure nausea and lethargy. It was also considered to be a nerve tonic, a relaxant and to counteract melancholy. It has been used for some skin and respiratory problems, for those with 'giddiness in the head' and tinnitus, and as a remedy for insect bites. It was also a remedy to counteract the effects of taking too much opium.

Medicinal discoveries Attention has focused on the use of feverfew for treating migraines. Scientific studies show feverfew preparations to have anti-inflammatory and pain-relieving properties. Studies in migraine sufferers have shown that leaf preparations might help prevent migraine attacks. Feverfew has also been investigated for potential use in rheumatoid arthritis, although more studies are needed to confirm any benefits. Some people may have an allergic reaction after touching the plant.

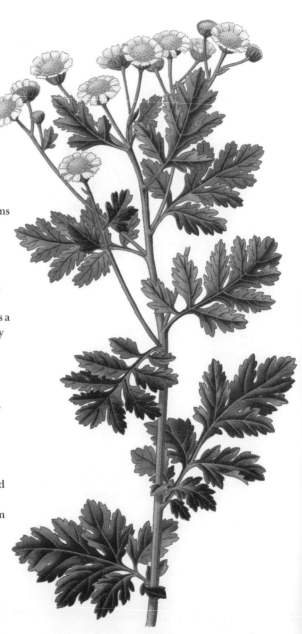

Taraxacum officinale
Dandelion, lion's tooth

Perennial native to the northern hemisphere and occurs as different subspecies with yellow flowers. Grows wild, often in meadows and along roadsides.

Part(s) used Aerial parts, root.

Traditional uses Taken to purify the blood, cleanse the body and aid elimination of toxins. It was also used as a gentle laxative and as a remedy to ease digestion, relieve gastric discomfort, stimulate the liver and improve appetite. It was regarded as a diuretic – in France it is known as 'pissenlit' ('wet-the-bed'). It was also considered a remedy for rheumatic complaints and skin conditions such as eczema, and the juice was painted on warts. In traditional Chinese medicine, it has been used for liver disorders, abscesses and snake bites.

Medicinal discoveries Modern uses of dandelion are based on some of the traditional uses. Dandelion preparations are taken to alleviate stomach and intestinal complaints, including flatulence. Some scientific studies suggest that herb preparations appear to have more effective diuretic properties compared to root preparations. The high potassium content of the plant is considered to contribute to the diuretic effects. Other studies suggest dandelion root has anti-inflammatory properties. Some individuals may have an allergic reaction after touching the plant.

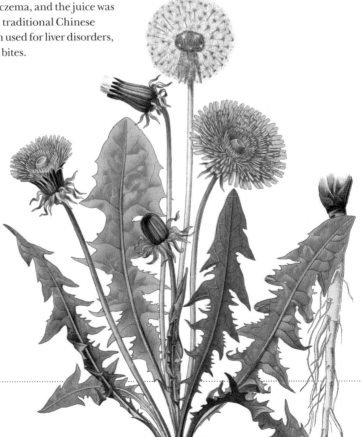

Terminalia chebula
Terminalia

Medium to large deciduous tree native to S. Asia. Produces unpleasant-smelling, white-yellow flowers in late spring. Nut-like fruits are yellow to orange-brown. Can be grown as an ornamental in a large garden.

Part(s) used Fruit.
Traditional uses Has multiple uses in Ayurvedic and Tibetan medicines to treat asthma, bile duct disorders, insect stings, sore throat, hiccups, diarrhoea, dysentery, bleeding piles, ulcers, gout, vomiting and heart and bladder diseases.
Medicinal discoveries There is some scientific data to support its use for the treatment of cardiovascular problems.

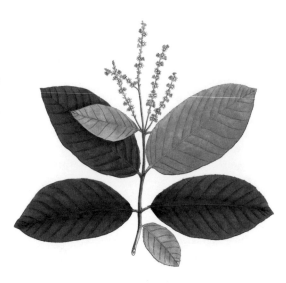

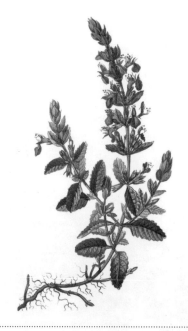

Teucrium chamaedrys
Germander

An evergreen shrub from Europe and S.W. Asia with miniature, oak-shaped, aromatic leaves and purple summer flowers. Found growing on rocky outcrops and old walls.

Part(s) used Aerial parts.
Traditional uses The herbalist Culpeper (see page 81) claimed the plant was a remedy for melancholy, headaches, convulsions and drowsiness. It was also reputed to alleviate coughs and asthma, and was applied for skin problems and snake bites.
Medicinal discoveries Preparations have shown antimicrobial and antioxidant properties. However, there are reports that suggest *Teucrium* species may cause liver damage.

Thymus vulgaris
Garden thyme

A hardy, evergreen, cushion-forming shrub native to the Mediterranean. Produces white to pink-purple flowers in late spring to early summer. Foliage is highly aromatic.

Part(s) used Flower, leaf.

Traditional uses Taken as a pungent and warming remedy to aid chills and lethargy and to lift the spirits. Thyme was used to relieve spasms, for flatulence and to stimulate digestion and help the appetite. It was considered to act as a diuretic, as an antiseptic for urine infections and as a treatment for intestinal worms. It was applied to the skin to ease joint pains and used as an antiseptic mouthwash and gargle to soothe inflammation. Thyme has also been used as an expectorant and cough remedy. *Thymus serpyllum* (creeping thyme) was an ancient remedy for hangovers.

Medicinal discoveries Thyme contains an essential oil and flavonoid components that are considered to contribute to the antispasmodic, antiseptic, expectorant and cough-relieving effects of the plant. The herb is taken as an infusion, considered to alleviate symptoms of bronchitis, catarrhs and respiratory infections. Scientific studies have associated thyme with antibacterial and antifungal effects. It was also shown to help treat intestinal worms. Other studies suggest thyme might help reduce pain, inflammation and fevers. Thyme contains compounds with antioxidant properties.

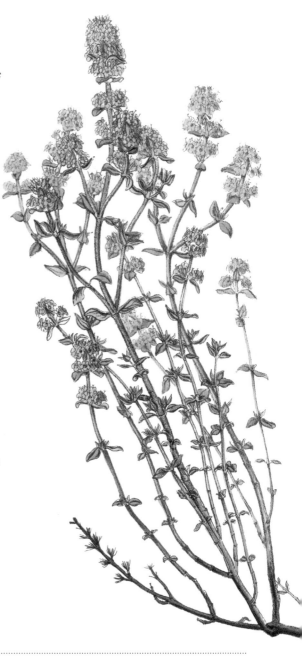

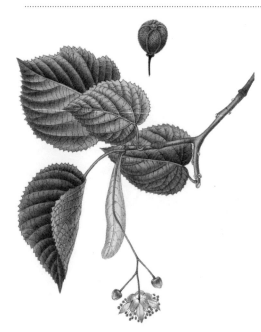

Tilia x *europaea*
Common lime, linden

Deciduous tree native to Europe. Dark green, heart-shaped leaves with fragrant yellow flowers in early summer. A popular street tree, despite its susceptibility to aphids that produce a sticky honeydew which is deposited on anything under the tree.

Part(s) used Flower.
Traditional uses Used as a tea since the Middle Ages to promote perspiration to break fevers and as a gentle sedative to treat nervous disorders. Still used for colds, fevers and headaches.
Medicinal discoveries Scientific studies show extracts have anti-inflammatory properties.

Toxicodendron quercifolium
Poison ivy

Shrub native to N. America. Vine-like plant with oak-like leaves and small green-yellow flowers in summer. The sap from the plant can cause severe allergic reactions.

Part(s) used Leaf.
Traditional uses Alcoholic tinctures used in remedies for rheumatism, ringworm and other skin disorders. In eighteenth-century Britain it was prescribed for persistent herpes sores and palsy. Later used to treat paralysis, acute rheumatism and pain relief.
Medicinal discoveries Poison ivy contains the compound urushiol, which can cause serious skin problems. The plant also contains flavonols, which could explain some of its traditional applications.

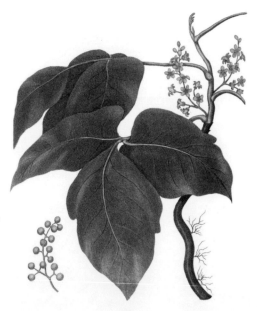

Tragopogon porrifolius
Salsify, oyster plant

Mediterranean biennial with green-blue
leaves and pink-purple flowers in summer.

Part(s) used Root, shoot.
Traditional uses Both the roots and shoots
of salsify have been cultivated for food. In
Lebanese folk medicine they were also used
as a remedy for liver problems and cancer.
Medicinal discoveries Studies suggest
that aerial parts of the plant have anti-
inflammatory properties. The plant has
also been investigated for antioxidant,
anticancer and liver-protective effects and
for its potential to lower cholesterol, reduce
appetite and counteract fatigue.

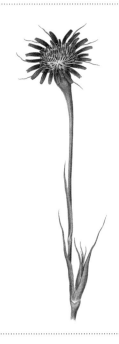

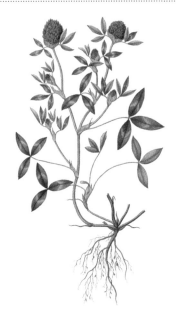

Trifolium pratense
Red clover, trefoil

European perennial now naturalized widely
in meadows and grassed areas. From early
summer to autumn it produces pink-purple
flowers. Grown as a fodder crop.

Part(s) used Flower.
Traditional uses Used to treat skin complaints,
particularly eczema and psoriasis, and was
reputed to relax spasms. It was also used as
an expectorant and diuretic.
Medicinal discoveries Red clover contains
compounds called isoflavones that have
oestrogen-like effects. Modern interest in
red clover has focused on its potential to
reduce menopausal symptoms and some
studies suggest it might help alleviate
symptoms such as hot flushes.

Trigonella foenum-graecum
Fenugreek

Annual Mediterranean herb with lush, light green foliage and small, white flowers in early summer, followed, in autumn, by long, thin seed pods. Grows in most soils but needs sun.

Part(s) used Seed.
Traditional uses Used as a carminative, a gastric stimulant, to induce lactation and as an antidiabetic. In Europe it was taken to improve appetite and soothe inflamed skin.
Medicinal discoveries The plant contains compounds with anti-inflammatory and antimicrobial properties. These properties may also inhibit cancerous cells in the liver and reduce cholesterol levels.

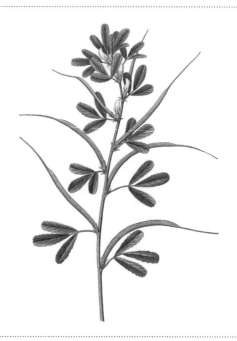

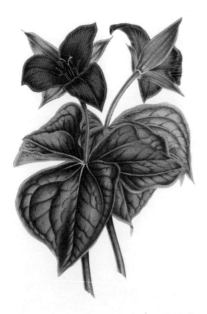

Trillium erectum
Beth root, birth root

Perennial native to N. American woods and forests. Erect stems bear diamond-shaped leaves, with nodding deep maroon or white flowers in spring. Grows in moist but well-drained soils in deep or partial shade.

Part(s) used Root.
Traditional uses Native Americans used the plant as a woman's herb to aid childbirth. It was also used as a tonic and antiseptic to treat skin problems.
Medicinal discoveries The steroidal saponins in the root could explain the use of the plant in childbirth. Further research is needed to support its use as an antiseptic.

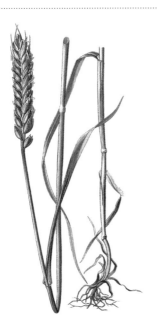

Triticum aestivum
Bread wheat

Annual thought to be originally from the Middle East, bread wheat was domesticated at least 9,000 years ago and today there are about 5,000 cultivars. The ear contains the flowering and fruiting parts.

Part(s) used Aerial parts.
Traditional uses Oil was used in antimicrobial treatments, for kidney and urinary tract infections. Extracts of aerial parts were used in cough remedies, as a sedative and to treat night sweats, sore throats and muscle pain.
Medicinal discoveries Extracts have antibacterial activity and can lower blood cholesterol and decrease lipids in liver tissue.

Turnera diffusa
Damiana

Aromatic perennial shrub that grows in dry, sandy, rocky areas of Central and S. America. It has yellow-orange summer flowers.

Part(s) used Leaf, stem.
Traditional uses In S. America it was taken to improve libido, and for nervous conditions, including anxiety and depression. It was taken as a laxative and stimulant, and to alleviate menstrual and menopausal problems. Damiana is brewed as a tea and is used to flavour liqueurs.
Medicinal discoveries Tests suggest damiana might reduce blood sugar, so is of interest for its potential use in diabetes. It has antibacterial properties and has been investigated for its effects on bladder infections.

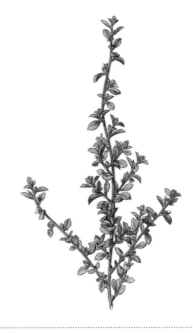

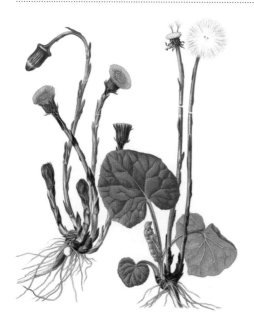

Tussilago farfara
Coltsfoot

Creeping perennial with dandelion-like yellow flowers. Found on uncultivated ground in Europe, Asia and N. Africa; introduced to N. America.

Part(s) used Flower, leaf.
Traditional uses Used as an expectorant and to soothe coughs. Leaves were smoked as a 'herbal tobacco' to alleviate catarrh, asthma and bronchitis. They were also used as a decoction for asthma and colds.
Medicinal discoveries Coltsfoot has been investigated for anti-blood clotting activity and anti-inflammatory and antibacterial properties. It contains pyrrolizidine alkaloids which are associated with liver damage.

Typha latifolia
Bulrush, cat's tail

Aquatic perennial with poker-like, brown flower spikes. Often planted in ponds as an ornamental. Can be invasive and is considered a weed in parts of Australia.

Part(s) used Fruiting spike produced following pollination, pollen.
Traditional uses Pollen was used for bleeding disorders following injuries. It was also used for menstruation pain and abscesses; it was reputed to have diuretic properties, aid circulation and be a remedy for diarrhoea. The fruit was used in N. America as a traditional remedy for burns and wounds.
Medicinal discoveries Studies suggest that fruit preparations have some properties that might promote wound healing.

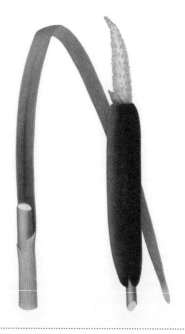

Plant compounds

Unlike animals, plants are usually fixed in one place so they cannot escape from danger by running away or travel to find a mate. During the evolutionary process they developed other survival and reproductive strategies, such as enzyme systems, to enable them to synthesize complex compounds to deal with challenges from their environment and successfully compete for living space and nutrients.

Some of these plant compounds are brightly coloured, such as the flavonoids that occur in flowers and berries. There are over 2,000 types of flavonoids, which include flavones that are often yellow, such as in yarrow (*Achillea millefolium*) flowers, and anthocyanins that can be blue, such as those in cornflowers (*Cyanus segetum*), or red, such as in rose (*Rosa* species) petals. These 'colouring' compounds also help to attract pollinators, such as bees, enabling transfer of pollen. Birds are attracted to brightly coloured berries as a source of food, which helps seed dispersal. Pollination and seed dispersal are important strategies for the survival of plant species.

Many flavonoids have antioxidant properties, which help protect plants from the damaging effects of free radicals from exposure to sun (UV) light. Plants also produce compounds to stop them freezing in cold climates. In drought conditions, mucilage compounds (carbohydrates), such as in *Aloe vera* gel, help to preserve moisture.

Other plant compounds, such as monoterpenes, have fragrant odours and attract pollinators or deter predators. Monoterpenes occur in many plant oils, such as lavender (*Lavandula* species) oil, which we are familiar with as essential oils used in aromatherapy. Some plant compounds, including monoterpenes in thyme (*Thymus* species) oil, have antimicrobial properties, which help protect plants from disease.

To prevent them from being eaten by predators, some plants produce toxic compounds (many are alkaloids) that act as warning chemicals and poisons. Some poisonous plants, including deadly nightshade (*Atropa belladonna*) and mandrake (*Mandragora officinarum*) produce toxic alkaloids, such as hyoscyamine and hyoscine, which, although poisonous to predators and humans, have also been developed as useful pharmaceuticals.

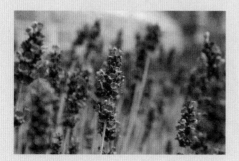

Aerial parts of lavender (*Lavandula* species) contain fragrant compounds, including monoterpenes, which may attract pollinators or deter predators.

Urtica dioca
Stinging nettle

The stinging action of the nettle, which is the bane of many a gardener, was considered a boon by Roman soldiers who brought the plant with them to Britain. To make the harsh winters more bearable they would sting themselves with the plant to increase circulation. Nettles are sometimes used in a similar way today by the brave to relieve arthritis pain, an action known as rubefacient, or counter-irritant.

Although nettles produce a strong allergic reaction externally, internally they act as an anti-inflammatory for allergic conditions. A tea of nettle leaf, elderflower and plantain is a traditional remedy for hayfever, and nettles are also recommended by herbalists for asthma and eczema. Nettle leaves have been taken as a diuretic, for gout, and to control blood sugar. Small studies show nettle roots can reduce urinary symptoms of benign prostate hyperplasia (enlarged prostate gland).

The Roman poet Ovid includes the seeds in a recipe for an aphrodisiac drink, and as with other aphrodisiacs, nettle is considered a tonic to improve general health and resilience. Leaves are rich in antioxidant vitamins A, C and E, the minerals magnesium, calcium and iron and B vitamins. They are also relatively high in fibre.

Grow Fast growing. Grows in rich, moist soil. Plant in a container to stop it spreading.
Harvest Wear thick gloves! Pick before flowering and take only the top four to six leaves.
Caution Nettles can aggravate the gut if picked when in flower.

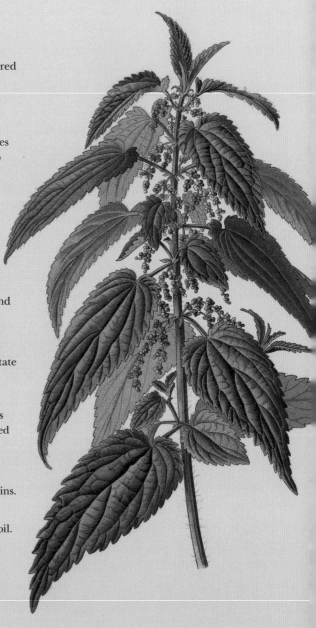

Nettle soup

The nutritional benefits of nettles can be enjoyed in this classic soup. When handling the fresh leaves, protect your fingers from stings by wearing rubber gloves.

½ an onion, finely chopped

Knob of butter

2 dried bay leaves

700 ml (24 fl oz) vegetable or chicken stock

1 small potato, diced

100 g (3½ oz) stinging nettles, rinsed

1 clove of garlic, crushed

Handful of fresh sage, rosemary or thyme, chopped

1. In a heavy-based saucepan, fry the onion and bay leaves in a knob of butter until soft.

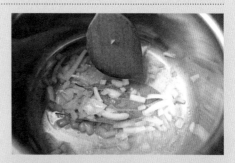

2. Add the stock and potatoes, cover the pan and cook until the potatoes are soft. Reduce the heat and stir in the nettles, garlic and herbs. Cook for a further five minutes.

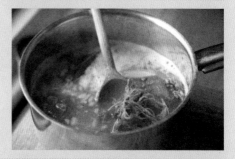

3. Remove the bay leaves. Blend the soup and serve. If you like, add a swirl of cream to each bowl of soup.

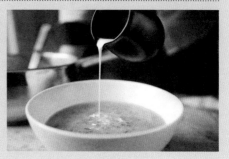

Vaccinium myrtillus
Common bilberry

Deciduous, low-growing shrub found on acid soils in woodland and heathland in N. Europe. Flowers in early summer with blue-black fruit in the autumn.

Part(s) used Flower, fruit, leaf.
Traditional uses Flowers were used for eye problems, cancer, diabetes and circulatory and gastrointestinal tract disorders. Flower-based herbal supplements were used for circulatory problems, and to improve vision, lower blood glucose and to treat diarrhoea.

Medicinal discoveries Bilberries are a rich source of anthocyanins, the pigments which give the fruits their blue-black colour and their high antioxidant activity. These compounds have been reported to lower blood glucose and to have anti-inflammatory and lipid-lowering effects. Experiments have shown they lower oxidative stress which contributes to the use of bilberry for cancer, diabetes and cardiovascular disease, as well as dementia and other age-related diseases. A commercial anthocyanin-rich extract from bilberry was shown in laboratory studies to inhibit the growth of colon cancer cells without affecting the growth of normal colon cells. This suggests a possible specific action against cancer cells and justification for further research.

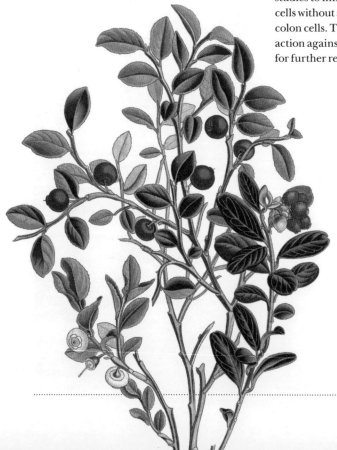

Drugs from plants

In the nineteenth century, the pain-relieving chemicals morphine and codeine were isolated from opium, the latex of the opium poppy (*Papaver somniferum*). In the same century, the antimalarial drug quinine was isolated from *Cinchona* bark. These discoveries revolutionized the development of medicines, leading to a new era that involved the isolation of single chemicals from plants with pharmacological properties, and formulating the active constituent, or 'drug', as a medicine. Today, morphine, codeine and quinine are still important medicines and knowledge of their chemical and medicinal properties enabled the design of other new medicines.

Plants have provided us with many key drugs. The alkaloids, vincristine and vinblastine, from the Madagascar periwinkle (*Catharanthus roseus*) are important medicines for some types of cancer. Another unique anticancer compound, paclitaxel, was discovered in Pacific yew (*Taxus brevifolia*) bark. Related compounds in the leaves of the common yew (*Taxus baccata*) were chemically modified in the laboratory to produce a more sustainable source of paclitaxel and new anticancer drugs. Other important drugs from plants include galantamine from toxic snowdrop (*Galanthus nivalis*) and daffodil (*Narcissus* species) bulbs, which is used to treat Alzheimer's disease symptoms, and digoxin from poisonous foxgloves (*Digitalis* species) used for some heart disorders. Plant chemicals can be modified in the laboratory to produce even better pharmaceuticals. For example, the discovery of cocaine from *Erythroxylum coca* leaves transformed surgical procedures in the 1800s and led to the development of modern anaesthetic drugs.

In modern medicine, about 40 per cent of pharmaceutical drugs are of natural origin. We still rely on plants to obtain some important drugs such as morphine and digoxin, as they cannot be synthesized from scratch in the laboratory. Plants are marvellous synthetic chemists and produce a host of diverse and complex chemicals, many of which may never have been discovered using synthetic chemistry routes. Plants remain a potential source of many other useful pharmaceuticals yet to be discovered.

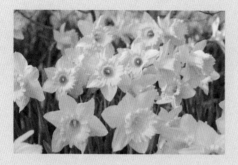

Daffodil (*Narcissus* species) bulbs contain the alkaloid galantamine, which has been developed as a drug to alleviate symptoms in Alzheimer's disease.

Valeriana officinalis
Valerian

Valerian is principally used as a sedative, helping to reduce and relieve anxiety, and for its hypnotic effect, improving the ability to fall asleep and the quality of sleep. These actions have been widely studied and valerian extracts have been shown to affect chemical messages in the brain that reduce stimulating nerve signals.

This effective 'slowing of the mind' supports the traditional use for those who are prone to worry. As this action is similar to the way benzodiazepine tranquilizers work, valerian is being investigated to help with withdrawal from these commonly prescribed medications. It may also explain valerian's traditional use for epilepsy. Essential oil of valerian was used to treat epilepsy in medieval Iranian medicine, while the root was widely seen as the best anti-epileptic medication available at the turn of the nineteenth century in Europe.

Valerian root is an ingredient in commercial sleep aid teas, often alongside other soporific herbs such as chamomile, lavender and hops. Herbalists today also use valerian as an antispasmodic to reduce muscular tension, gut spasms and menstrual cramps.

Grow A tall perennial found in the wild in woods, grassland and scrub on damp soil. Produces a tangle of fine roots: to make them easier to harvest grow in a container.
Harvest Remove the plant from its pot in autumn and cut away a portion of the roots.
Caution Can cause drowsiness so do not take if driving or operating machinery.

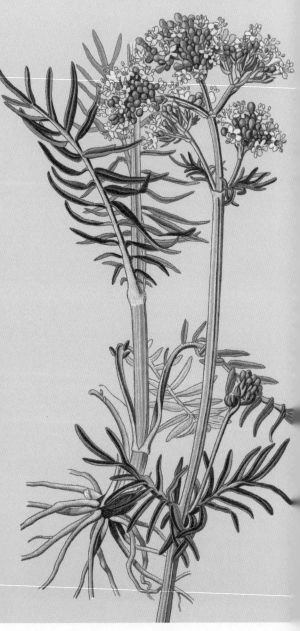

Dried valerian root

This drying method will work for other roots, although larger ones need to be sliced into small thin strips first. You can also use a dehydrator to dry them more quickly. Dried roots can then be made into teas, tinctures, syrups or powders.

Freshly dug valerian roots

You will also need: vegetable brush; wire drying rack; dehydrator (optional); brown paper bags; airtight storage jars or plastic food containers

1. Scrub the roots clean and pat dry with a clean teatowel.

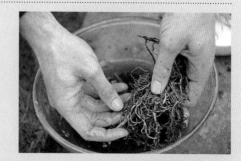

2. Spread the roots out on the drying rack in a single layer. Place in a warm dry place but out of direct sunlight.

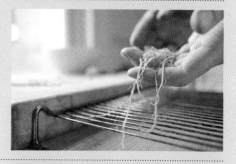

3. Leave until the roots feel dry and slightly brittle. Store in brown paper bags in airtight jars or plastic food containers in a cool place away from direct sunlight.

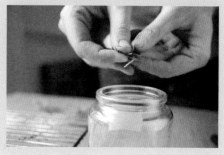

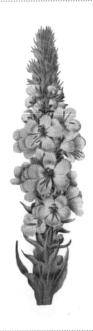

Verbascum densiflorum
Dense-flowered mullein

Biennial native to Europe with down-covered leaves and large spikes of showy, often yellow, cup-shaped flowers in summer. Most mulleins prefer sunny sites and grow best in well-drained soil.

Part(s) used Aerial parts.
Traditional uses Used for their antiseptic, astringent, demulcent, emollient and expectorant properties. An infusion was also used to treat various respiratory complaints including coughs, bronchitis, asthma and throat irritations.
Medicinal discoveries More scientific data is needed to confirm its traditional uses.

Verbascum thapsus
Common mullein, Aaron's rod

Biennial native to Europe and temperate Asia. It produces a tall spike of yellow flowers from a large rosette of woolly, grey-green leaves. Prefers full sun on poor, well-drained soils; on rich soils it will need support.

Part(s) used Flower, leaf, root.
Traditional uses Historically used for its demulcent, emollient and astringent properties. Tinctures from the whole plant are said to have mild sedative properties. The leaves and flowers were used for treating chest, lung and bowel problems. A poultice for hemorrhoids was made from the leaves.
Medicinal discoveries Oil from the flowers has antioxidant properties and is of interest for treating respiratory and skin problems.

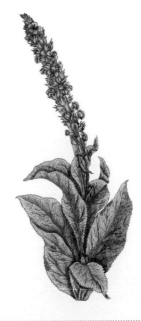

Verbena officinalis
Verbena, vervain

Upright perennial with white, pink or lilac
flowers. Found growing in temperate zones,
including E. Europe, often in hedgerows
and on wasteland.

Part(s) used Aerial parts.
Traditional uses Verbena was regarded
by the druids as a sacred herb. It was
used in magic and love potions and was
associated with witchcraft and sorcery.
In folk medicine, it was used as a diuretic,
to alleviate rheumatic complaints and
to promote lactation (milk production).
It was also taken as a tonic and as a remedy
for melancholia, stress, anxiety, headaches
and seizures. It was said to aid convalescence
after fevers and was taken for coughs
and colds. It was a topical treatment for
abrasions, burns and bites.
Medicinal discoveries Scientific studies show
verbena preparations and some constituents
of the plant have anti-inflammatory
properties. Other studies suggest verbena
might influence the actions of some
hormones, perhaps explaining its
reputation to stimulate lactation. Research
also shows it may have sedative properties
and might help protect nerve cells. Vervain
may have antiviral effects, and it might aid
the immune system and reduce coughs.
These actions might explain the traditional
use to aid recovery after fevers.

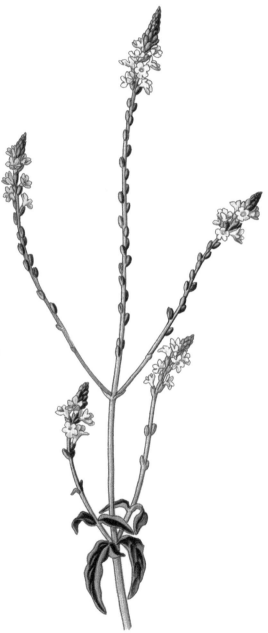

Veronica officinalis
Common speedwell

Perennial found growing across Europe.
It produces blue-lilac flowers in summer.

Part(s) used Aerial parts.
Traditional uses Used as an expectorant to
alleviate symptoms in bronchitis and asthma.
In cases of gout and rheumatism, it was made
into tea as a remedy for inflamed joints. It
was applied topically to aid wound healing,
stop itching and reduce foot perspiration.
Medicinal discoveries As a herbal medicine,
speedwell is still used as an appetite
stimulant and for conditions including
respiratory and gastrointestinal complaints
and arthritis. Scientific studies suggest the
herb has anti-inflammatory properties.

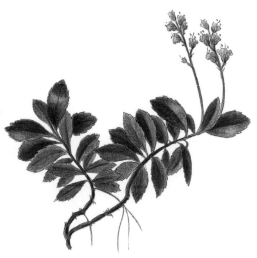

Viburnum prunifolium
Black haw, American sloe

Deciduous shrub native to N. America and
widely cultivated in the U.S. and Europe.
It produces small, white flowers in spring,
followed by blue-black berries.

Part(s) used Root bark and stem bark.
Traditional uses A traditional remedy for
period pain, for spasms and asthma. It
was reputed to prevent miscarriage and to
alleviate vomiting in pregnancy and the
symptoms of the menopause.
Medicinal discoveries Some scientific studies
suggest black haw might help reduce spasms
of the uterus and the intestine. Other studies
suggest black haw might have beneficial
effects on the veins, although it has also been
linked with increasing blood pressure.

Conservation and trade

It is difficult to evaluate accurately the volume or value of the medicinal plant trade. It is known, however, that demand for many species is increasing and that this can lead to problems. One factor that makes gathering the data difficult is that a high proportion of medicinal plants are still harvested in the wild by local people. Many of these plants face increasing pressures from being over-harvested due to increased demand, changes in land use and failure due to environmental factors such as late frosts, droughts, flooding and problems with pollination.

It is important that medicinal plants are harvested sustainably, but when demand is high opportunists will often go into an area and lift all the plants. Monitoring this type of behaviour is difficult, although advances in diagnostic techniques now enable the origin of plants to be traced.

One solution is to cultivate the plants, but this is not always a straightforward solution: wild plants aren't always easy to grow and there is evidence that some material from cultivated plants does not have the efficacy of material harvested from the wild. The compounds in the plant associated with the medicinal properties might have a defence role in the plant's ecology; if the plant no longer needs to protect itself because it is treated with pesticides, then the level of the medicinal compounds in the plant may decrease.

Botanic gardens and gardeners can play an important role in plant conservation by propagating plants and saving seeds. In many parts of the world there is increased interest in conserving locally important plants.

Not all medicinal plants are threatened. Indeed, some examples listed in this book are classified as weeds, including couch grass (*Elymus repens*). Care should be taken when growing plants that are potentially invasive; if they escape from the confines of the garden they can compete with native species.

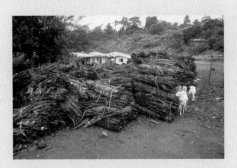

African cherry (*Prunus africana*) is threatened by over harvesting of the bark to make herbal medicine (see page 155)

Viola odorata
Sweet violet

In the *Trotula*, a book on women's medicine written in the twelfth century in Salerno, Italy, violets are recommended for 'excessive flux of the menses' and to extinguish heat in acute diseases by anointing the oil on the area of the liver, pulse points, temples, palms of the hand and soles of the feet. Violets are regularly seen as 'cooling' in their effect and used to treat heat or dryness.

Sixteenth-century herbalist John Gerard (see page 81) says of violet syrup, made from the flowers, as having 'power to ease inflammation, roughness of the throat and comforteth the heart, assuageth the pains of the head and causeth sleep'. He also recommended the juice or syrup for inflamed lungs, cough, fever and sore throat.

Although sweet violet appears regularly in old herbals, often with extensive descriptions, its use seems to have fallen out of favour in recent times. When it does appear, it is usually considered as a flower or leaf remedy for skin problems, in particular eczema, and for sore throats, coughs and catarrh. Its relative *Viola tricolor* (heartsease) is more widely used, often for the same conditions.

Grow Evergreen perennial. Plant in full sun to partial shade in moist, well-drained soil. Flowers in spring and in mild winters.
Harvest Pick flowers on a dry day when they are at their most fragrant.

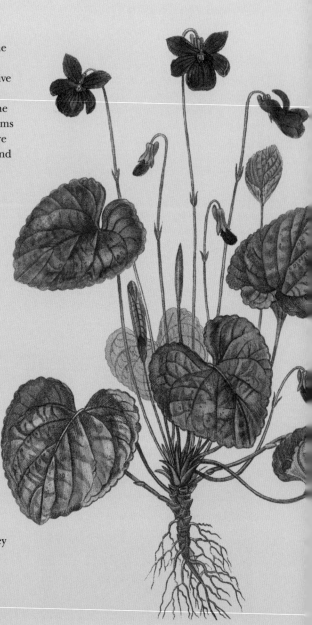

Sweet violet syrup

The syrup is traditionally used for a sore throat or cough. To achieve a more purple hue add lemon juice drop by drop. Take a teaspoon of syrup three times a day.

3 handfuls freshly picked sweet violets

Caster sugar

Half a lemon, juice only

You will also need: saucepan; sieve; measuring jug; spoon; sterilized bottles with stoppers

1. Put the flowers in a saucepan and add sufficient water to just cover them.

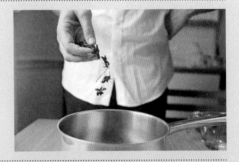

2. Heat gently until the water just begins to simmer. Remove from the heat, cover with a tight-fitting lid and leave overnight.

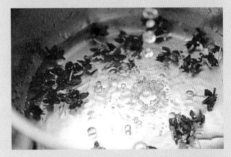

3. Strain the liquid through a sieve into a measuring jug. For each 30 ml (1 fl oz) of liquid add 30 g (1 oz) of sugar. Pour the mixture back into a saucepan and dissolve the sugar over a gentle heat, stirring continuously. Pour into sterilized bottles. If you wish to enhance the purple colour of the syrup, add lemon juice drop by drop. Store in a cool dark place, will keep for one year.

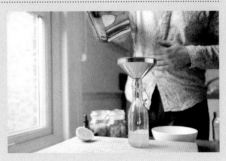

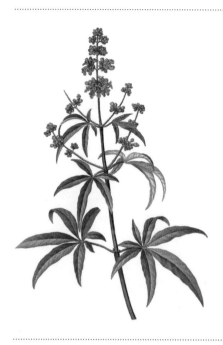

Vitex agnus-castus
Chastetree, agnus-castus

Deciduous shrub from S. Europe. Grows in well-drained soils in full sun. Has clusters of purple flowers that bloom in late summer. Similar leaf shape to cannabis.

Part(s) used Aerial parts.
Traditional uses Used to treat menstrual irregularities, premenstrual syndrome and the menopause. Also used for acne, nervousness, dementia, joint conditions, colds, upset stomach, spleen disorders, headaches, migraine, eye pain, inflammation and swellings.
Medicinal discoveries A clinical study on patients showed a significant reduction in premenstrual syndrome symptoms. Still used for menstrual problems.

Vitis vinifera
Grape

Deciduous, climbing vine native to Asia. Yellow flowers occur in clusters and plants produce fruit from the second year. Grows in most soils but requires warm conditions.

Part(s) used Fruit, leaf.
Traditional uses Leaves used to staunch bleeding, reduce inflammation and ease pain. Unripe grapes were used to treat sore throats; dried grapes were taken for constipation, cancer, cholera, smallpox, nausea, eye infections, and skin, kidney and liver diseases.
Medicinal discoveries Still used for many conditions but scientific data are lacking to support many of these traditional uses.

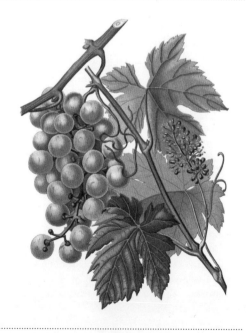

Withania somnifera
Ashwagandha, Indian ginseng

Perennial that grows in India, Africa and
the Mediterranean.

Part(s) used Root, fruit, leaf.
Traditional uses A rejuvenative tonic in
Ayurvedic medicine, for convalescence and
old age. It was taken to regain youth, aid
memory and intellect, protect against diseases,
as an aphrodisiac and to help the body cope
with stress.
Medicinal discoveries Modern interest has
focused on use of the root for memory problems
such as Alzheimer's disease. Scientific studies
show root preparations improve learning and
memory and may help protect nerve cells.
They are anti-inflammatory so of interest to
alleviate arthritis.

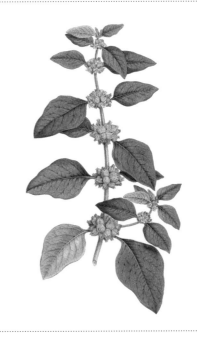

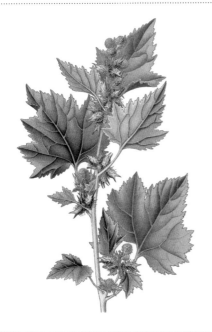

Xanthium strumarium
Cocklebur

Green-flowering annual often considered
a weed. The fruit is covered with prickles.

Part(s) used Fruit.
Traditional uses Taken to ease the pain of
rheumatic complaints and combat leprosy.
A traditional Chinese medicine reputed to
counteract allergic conditions and itching
and to relieve catarrhs.
Medicinal discoveries Studies suggest fruit
preparations have anti-inflammatory
properties which may help alleviate
symptoms in arthritis. Some constituents of
the fruit might alleviate symptoms in allergic
rhinitis, others may cause liver damage.
Leaf preparations have antibacterial and
antioxidant properties.

Zea mays
Sweet corn, maize

Annual grass from S. America or Mexico with attractive bamboo-like foliage and yellow flowers that develop into edible seed cobs. The corn varies in colour depending on the variety.

Part(s) used Corn silk (stamens), fruit, leaf.
Traditional uses Wide range of traditional uses. Cobs were ground to make a poultice to treat bruises, swellings, sores and headaches. They were also used to make a tincture to expel excess fluids from the body. Corn silk was used as a soothing diuretic and to treat acute inflammation and irritations of the urinary system. It was also used to reduce blood pressure and relieve symptoms associated with gout and arthritis.

Medicinal discoveries Corn, which has antibacterial properties, has been added to toothpastes, mouthwashes and oral hygiene products. Research has shown that saponins and allantoin in the leaves and cobs have anti-inflammatory properties and promote wound healing. These compounds could explain the other uses of corn.

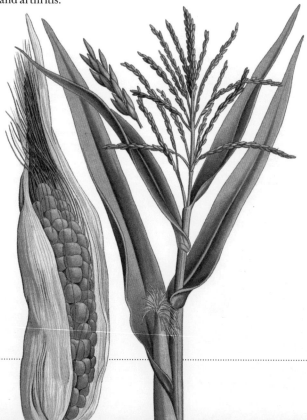

Zingiber officinale
Ginger

Ginger is considered native to S.E. Asia and grows well at subtropical temperatures with good rainfall. Plants are cultivated in many regions, including India, China, Australia and tropical parts of the US such as Florida. Ginger is grown in the same way as the potato: rhizomes with buds are planted in nutrient-rich, well-drained loam.

Part(s) used Rhizome.

Traditional uses Ginger has been cultivated in India since ancient times as a flavouring, and for its warming and invigorating properties. It is thought to calm the digestive system, to stimulate sweating and help with fevers. It has been used to treat digestive problems, such as colic and heartburn, and the problems associated with flatulence.

Medicinal discoveries Ginger is used as a herbal remedy to prevent nausea and vomiting, including travel sickness, to aid digestion and to alleviate inflamed joints, such as in rheumatoid arthritis. Scientific studies suggest ginger has anti-inflammatory, anti-ulcer and anti-sickness properties, although more studies are needed to confirm these effects. The pungency of ginger is attributed to the essential oil content. The oil and resin mixture from the rhizomes, the 'oleo-resin', and other rhizome preparations have shown some promising effects in reducing cholesterol levels.

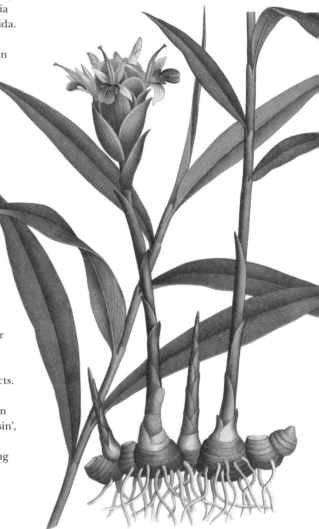

Glossary

Acetylcholinesterase An enzyme that occurs within the nervous system, which degrades the chemical messenger acetylcholine

Adaptogen A substance that aids non-specific resistance to adverse influences, such as stress and disease

Aerial parts All the component parts of a plant that appear above the roots

Alkaloid A type of compound synthesised by plants that contains nitrogen in its chemical structure; alkaloids often have a marked physiological effect on humans and animals

Analgesic A substance that can relieve pain

Annual Plant that completes its lifecycle from germination, flowering to setting seed and dying back in one growing year

Anthocyanin A sub-class of flavonoid synthesised by plants; anthocyanins are the pigments often responsible for the blue, purple and red colours of flowers

Anthraquinone A type of compound synthesised by plants; anthraquinones often have cathartic properties

Anthrone A type of compound synthesised by plants; anthrones are derivatives of anthraquinones

Antiarrhythmic Combats arrhythmias (irregular heartbeats)

Anticoagulant Prevents coagulation (of blood)

Antipyretic Reduces fever

Antispasmodic Prevents or alleviates muscle spasms (cramps)

Antitrypanosomal Antiparasitic against *Trypanosoma* species, which are parasites that can infect the blood of vertebrates, including humans

Arteriosclerosis Hardening of the arteries (blood vessels)

Astringent Causes shrinkage of tissues, arrests secretions or controls bleeding

Benign prostatic hyperplasia Enlargement of the prostate (not usually associated with cancer)

Benzylisoquinoline alkaloid A class of alkaloid synthesised by plants such as poppies

Biennial Plant that usually completes its lifecycle in two growing years, producing foliage only in the first year then flowers and fruits in the second

Biliary Relating to bile

Biofilm A thin coating of microorganisms together with other substances such as proteins; often associated with coating the surface of teeth

Bract Modified leaf at the base of a flower

Calyx The collective term for sepals that form the outer whorl of a flower

Canavanine A non-protein amino acid that occurs in some plants, especially some legume seeds

Cardiac Pertaining to the heart

Cardiac glycoside Plant compound that has steroidal-type properties; cardiac glycosides may slow the heart

Cardiotonic Exerts a favourable action on the heart

Carminative A remedy that relieves flatulence

Cholera An infectious disease caused by the bacterium *Vibrio cholerae*; involves symptoms such as diarrhoea

Clinical study (clinical trial) A controlled study or experiment that involves a defined set of human subjects that receive a form of medical intervention (such as a medicine) to obtain scientifically valid information about the efficacy and safety of that medical intervention

Colitis Inflammation of the colon, a part of the large intestine

Coronary Denotes the coronary blood vessels of the heart

Coumarin A type of compound synthesised by plants, particularly by those in the bean family (Leguminosae)

Culpeper, Nicholas (1616–1654) English apothecary and physician who wrote and translated many medical books that integrated ideas from the Doctrine of Signatures and astrology into herbal medicine

Cyclic AMP Cyclic adenosine 3′,5′-cyclic monophosphate; formed in muscle and is a metabolic regulator

Deciduous Plant that sheds leaves annually at the end of the growing season

Decoction A preparation that involves boiling of a herbal drug in water prior to straining

Demulcent A substance that relieves irritation or inflammation, especially of mucous surfaces such as the throat

Dermatitis Inflammation of the skin

Dioscorides, Pedanius (40–90 AD) Greek physician and author of *De Materia Medica*, one of the most influential Western herbals of all time

Diphtheria An infectious disease caused by the bacterium *Corynebacterium diphtheriae* and its highly potent toxin

Diterpenoid A class of terpenoid compound synthesised by plants; the 'active' constituents' of some medicinal plants

Diuretic Promotes excretion of urine

Diverticulitis Inflammation of the diverticulum in the intestine

Dropsy Historical term for oedema (accumulation of fluid), often associated with heart failure

Dysentery A disease caused by an infection, which produces symptoms of watery diarrhoea and fever

Dyspepsia Disorder of the stomach that usually involves pain, nausea and indigestion

Emetic Causes vomiting

Emollient A substance that is applied to sooth or soften the skin

Evergreen Plant that retains leaves for more than one growing season

Expectorant Promotes the secretion of sputum (mucus) by the air passages, especially to treat coughs

Febrile Relates to fever

Febrifuge Reduces fever

Fibromyalgia A syndrome that involves widespread soft-tissue pain together with weakness, fatigue, aching and stiffness of affected muscles

Flavonoid A type of compound synthesised by plants and widely distributed in nature; flavonoids occur as different sub-classes and often have antioxidant properties

Gastritis Inflammation of the stomach

Gerard, John (1545–1612) English herbalist and gardener; author of *The Herball*, which included descriptions of over 1000 plant species

Gingivitis Inflammation of the gingiva (tissue that surrounds the neck of the teeth)

Glaucoma A disease that is characterised by increased pressure in the eye and leads to defects in the field of vision

Glycosides A plant compound that consists of two components: an aglycone (non-sugar) part and a sugar part

Gonorrhoea A contagious disease caused by the bacterium *Neisseria gonorrhoeae*, which causes inflammation of the genital region

Gynecological Pertaining to diseases of the female genital tract, associated with reproduction and hormonal factors

Haematuria Presence of blood in the urine

Hepatitis Inflammation of the liver

Hypertension High blood pressure

Hypertensive Denotes a person having high blood pressure

Immunosuppressive Prevention or interference with the development of an immune response

Infusion A preparation obtained by steeping a herbal drug in water

Iridoid A monoterpene type compound synthesised by plants; iridoids occur in some medicinal plants such as valerian and gentian

Isoflavone A sub-class of flavonoid compound synthesised by plants; isoflavones often have oestrogen-like properties

Isoquinoline alkaloid A class of alkaloid synthesised by plants such as poppies

Jaundice Increased levels of bile pigments in blood, causing a yellowish stain in some tissues of the body and in excretions

Latex A milky-white sap or fluid produced by some plants when the plant is cut or damaged; can be irritant

Lyme disease A bacterial infection spread to humans by infected ticks

Marrubiin A diterpenoid that occurs in *Marrubium vulgare*

Menorrhagia Excessively prolonged or profuse menstrual periods

Monoterpene A class of terpenoid compound synthesised by plants; monoterpenes often occur in plant essential oils

Mucilage Substance occurring in plants that is usually composed of carbohydrates (polysaccharides), which may act as a storage material, such as for water
Mucilagious Pertaining to muclilage

Neuralgic Pertaining to nerve pain
Oedema A condition characterised by an excess of watery fluid collecting in the cavities or tissues of the body

Pathogen Any microorganism, virus or other biological substance causing disease
Perennial Plant that lives for two years or longer, and once mature, flowers annually
Peristalsis The movement of the intestine, involving muscle contraction and relaxation, to propel the contents onwards through the digestive system
Phenolic A class of compound synthesised by plants that contains a phenol component in the chemical structure; phenolics may include simple acids, flavonoids, anthraquinones and coumarins
Phlebitis Inflammation of a vein
Placebo An inert substance given as a medicine for its suggestive effect; often included in clinical trials to compare with a drug substance under study
Pleurisy Inflammation of the pleura, which surround the lungs
Post-herpetic neuralgia Nerve pain that occurs following infection with the virus that causes shingles

Psoriasis A condition that involves inflamed and scaling lesions of the skin
Poultice A preparation formed by wetting an absorbent substance with fluids that may be medicated, which is applied to the skin to mediate an effect
Pulmonary Pertaining to the lungs
Pyrrolizidine alkaloid A class of alkaloid synthesised by plants; many have been associated with causing liver toxicity

Rheumatism Term used to describe various conditions associated with joint or muscle pain
Rhizomatous Pertaining to a rhizome
Rubefacient A substance that may alleviate pain by acting as a counter-irritant that produces erythema (reddening) when applied to the skin

Saponin A type of compound synthesised by plants; often associated with surfactant (detergent-like) properties
Scarlet fever A disease caused by a bacterial infection, which causes eruption of red lesions on the skin
Scrofula A disease with glandular swellings; historical term for tuberculosis
Sennoside A type of compound synthesised by plants; sennosides are the active components found in the laxative herb senna
Smallpox A contagious disease caused by the pox virus, causing

chills, fever and pustules on the skin; now considered eradicated due to vaccination programs
Soporific Causes or aids sleep
Stamen Male part of a flower
St Anthony's fire Refers to any of several inflammatory or gangrenous conditions of the skin
Stolon A horizontal spreading or arching stem that usually grows above ground and roots at its tip to produce a new plant
Stomachic A substance that improves appetite or digestion
Strewing herb Plants (often herbs) that were historically strewn over floors to provide fragrant odours, or to repel pests, in buildings
Tinnitus A condition involving the perception of sound, such as ringing or whistling noises in the ears
Triterpenoid A class of terpenoid compound synthesised by plants; abundant in nature, particularly in plant resins
Tuberculosis A disease caused by infection with the bacterium *Mycobacterium tuberculosis*, which can affect almost any tissue or organ of the body, such as the lungs
Turner, William (1508 - 1568) English botanist and naturalist

Uterotonic Gives tone to the uterine muscle

Vasodilative Causes dilation of blood vessels
Vitiligo A disorder that involves the appearance of non-pigmented patches on skin

Index

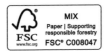

Picture acknowledgments

P33 Jan Kops et al. - Flora Batava - Permission granted to
use under GFDL by Kurt Stueber. Source: www.biolib.de
P47 Martin de Argenta, V., Album de la flora médico-
farmacéutica é industrial, indígena y exótica, vol. 2: t. 67
(1863) [I. Salcedo]
P50 Ruiz Lopez, H., Pavon, J.A., Flora Peruviana, et Chilensis,
Plates 153-325, vol. 2: p. 24, t. 245, fig. b (1798-1802)
P69 L'Héritier de Brutelle, C.L., Stirpes novae aut minus
cognitae, t. 78 (1784)
P71 Bessler, Basilius, Hortus Eystettensis, vol. 3: Quartus
ordo collectarum plantarum autumnalium, t. 360, fig. I (1620)
[B. Bessler]
P91 Siebold, P.F. von, Zuccarini, J.G., Flora Japonica,
t. 136 (1875)
P101 Bessler, Basilius, Hortus Eystettensis, vol. 2:
Quintus ordo collectarum plantarum aestivalium, t. 206
(1620) [B. Bessler]
P129 Jaume Saint-Hilaire, J.H., Traité des arbres forestiers,
t. 44 (1824)
P133 Blanco, M., Flora de Filipinas, t. 257 (1875)
P152 English botany, or coloured figures of British plants,
ed. 3 [B] [J.E. Sowerby et al], vol. 8: t. 1230 (1868)
P176 Plants of the coast of Coromandel vol. 1
(http://www.botanicus.org/page/280080),
William Roxburgh (1751-1815), Sir Joseph Banks (1743-1820)
P177 Getty images/Judy Unger
P186 Roxburgh, W., Plants of the coast of Coromandel,
vol. 1: t. 24 (1795) [n.a.]
P194 Roxburgh, W., Plants of the coast of Coromandel,
vol. 2: t. 197 (1798) [n.a.]